shiatsu for women

Ray Ridolfi and Susanne Franzen

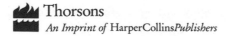

Thorsons
An Imprint of HarperCollinsPublishers

To the women in our professional and personal lives who have provided us with the information resource for this book.

Thorsons
An Imprint of HarperCollins*Publishers*
77–85 Fulham Palace Road
Hammersmith, London W6 8JB
1160 Battery Street
San Francisco, California 94111–1213

Published by Thorsons 1996

10 9 8 7 6 5 4 3 2 1

Ray Ridolfi and Susanne Franzen assert the moral right to be identified as the authors of this work

A catalogue record for this book
is available from the British Library

ISBN 1 85538 482 5

Text illustrations by Peter Cox

Printed and bound in Great Britain by
Scotprint Ltd, Musselburgh

contents

preface

Do you want to be a woman in charge of your own life, free from the restrictions of physical and emotional disturbances? You can be. Knowing how to prevent common illnesses and being able to control and speed your recovery from the physical and emotional stress of everyday life are just two of the many benefits you will gain from learning about shiatsu.

Shiatsu is a simple skill which you already have at your fingertips. It is 'touch' with a capital 'T'. As a woman, you may feel more comfortable expressing yourself through touch, and already be aware of how fulfilling the nurturing and caring expression of touching someone can be. For centuries, people have sought effective ways in which to help one another in times of need, and women have historically taken greater responsibility for caring for themselves, their children and partners in everyday life, particularly in times of illness. The medium of touch serves this purpose well. Touch has many different applications, such as in fear, anger, love, sympathy, compassion or desire. The intention behind the action is the important determining factor of the effect of the touch sensation.

More women than men come to us for individual shiatsu treatments and the student body of our shiatsu school is made up of approximately two thirds women, with 68 per cent of our graduate practitioners being women. We like to think that this enthusiasm demonstrates a more natural inclination and inherent ability for women to take responsibility for their own well-being. Add to this the enjoyment of touching and helping yourself and others, and you have the foundation for easily acquiring the basic skills of shiatsu.

You can develop this touch into a skilled and precise therapy, or simply use it to help yourself maintain good health and deal with some of those more common, persistent ailments which arise in life. No, it won't cure you of having an irritating bank manager – but it may change the way you react to them and many other sources of everyday stress.

Shiatsu is an Oriental medical therapy, a combination of physical techniques, diagnosis of signs and symptoms and a philosophical input. Thus, while it is substantially different from and yet similar in some ways to Western physiotherapy, shiatsu is more closely aligned to acupuncture philosophy and diagnostic theory. Many paramedically qualified professionals study shiatsu in order to enhance their understanding of the 'energetic' (the interaction between the physical and metaphysical body systems) and psycho-emotional relationships of the physical structure to the mind and emotions. If your aching premenstrual back is keeping you awake at night and making life a misery for you and everyone around you, then this is not just a 'physical' problem. It 'hurts' on all levels and life may seem pretty grey.

Shiatsu has a much wider effect than most people realize. Anyone working with shiatsu appreciates the emotional and physical strengthening that often occurs in the course of regular shiatsu treatments. Your physical appearance may seem more 'alive' and vibrant and you may even appear younger; these are certainly appreciated responses, although only perhaps the superficial physical reactions. There will be a much deeper effect on your consciousness and understanding of your place in the environment and society. It's what Buddhists call 'Big Mind' – a state of mind where the individual becomes aware of their place in the 'whole' of society and Nature, and how each action of the individual, no matter how small, effects the 'whole'. If everyone in the world could become more conscious of this relationship, it would be a healthier and happier place.

Shiatsu activates the natural self-healing mechanisms of your body to instigate a change to better health. This change may involve your body eliminating toxins and built-up emotions, which may or may not be a comfortable process. No two people are the same and therefore no two shiatsu treatments are the same. For this reason, we are only able to make general suggestions for self-treatment in this book, and the efficacy of any treatment suggestion may differ from person to person.

Preface

Some of the many benefits you will experience with shiatsu include:

- an improvement in your general health and well-being
- emotional and psychological balance
- relief from premenstrual tension
- a slowing down of the ageing process
- improved skin tone and more vital hair
- improved muscle flexibility and posture
- relief from stress and a calmer nervous system
- improved stamina
- enhanced libido and sexual enjoyment
- a more healthy pregnancy and childbirth

You have been practising the basics of shiatsu all your life. Touching, being touched, wanting to be touched and not wanting to be touched – it all depends on your mood and your 'approach'. Imagine that someone you like gives you a friendly bear hug. Do you melt with relaxation or is it the 'stiff upper lip' reaction where you grin and bear it? Touching and being touched becomes so relevant to your whole upbringing that maybe all touching is difficult and slightly 'taboo'. This is sad but true for many of us. Shiatsu is all about giving and receiving attention in a gentle and caring way. It makes you feel good. This is your opportunity to treat yourself with tender loving care, and give a bit of the same to others. Shiatsu offers an easy path to develop your natural abilities for self-health, even into a transforming and caring career. A saying we have in shiatsu is: 'Your shiatsu technique is only limited by your imagination.' *You* hold the key to unlocking your imagination. Will you let it free?

Finally, learning the techniques and philosophy of shiatsu takes time and practice. The bonus, however, is that the practice itself is already improving your health, both physically and mentally. You might like to learn all the interesting facts of Traditional Chinese Medicine (which talks of the Evil Pernicious Influences that penetrate your Defensive *Wei Ki* and injure your Life Force), or you may enjoy the Taoist philosophy of Yin and Yang in describing the wonder of Mother Nature and all phenomena. Maybe you don't give a hoot about any of these and just want to know how to reduce your period pains. All of these can be achieved through studying shiatsu. Shiatsu is user-friendly.

The Language in the Book

We have attempted to make the language in the book as clear as possible for both the complete beginner to shiatsu as well as the more experienced student or therapist. There are, however, a few instances which may need clarification.

When referring to the physical and energetic distinction between the organ and the function we have used, for example, 'liver' for the organ and 'Liver' for the energetic function.

Traditional Oriental Medical terminology, which adds both flavour and understanding to the information, is often juxtaposed with more common usage of language.

You will also find a glossary at the back containing some of the more commonly used terminology, to help you while you read.

Who Can Use this Book?

This is a user-friendly book containing basic information for self-assessment and treatment. Primarily aimed at women, it can be used for their partners in strengthening their relationship through touch communication. It will also be of use to students and practitioners of shiatsu to help deepen their knowledge for the treatment of women.

Please Note:

This book is not designed as a foundation for the diagnosis or treatment of any ailment without proper professional training. It is not intended as a replacement for medical advice or treatment, and the reader is advised to seek professional medical advice for any ailments.

PART I

chapter 1

Introducing Shiatsu

What Is Shiatsu?

Shiatsu is a contemporary bodywork therapy which works on all the different energetic levels of your body: physical, emotional and spiritual. It evolves from thousands of years of Oriental medical history and, specifically, from the traditional Japanese medical approach. 'Shiatsu' literally means 'finger pressure'. The actual treatment approach and philosophy are similar to those of acupuncture. Like acupuncture, shiatsu uses the 'meridians' (energy channels), 'tsubo' (pressure points) and comparable diagnostic methods, *but without the use of needles.* Unlike most other forms of bodywork, the receiver remains clothed for the treatment, and this is often a consideration for patients.

Describing shiatsu as 'finger pressure' is somewhat misleading, as the therapist will use their thumbs, hands, elbows, forearms, knees and sometimes feet during a treatment. Shiatsu acts upon the subtle anatomy of the body wherein energy known as 'Ki' flows to organs and all body areas through the pathways known as 'meridians'. These meridians are electromagnetic channels containing specific points of high electrical charge known as 'tsubo'. A combination of pressure point, meridian and body-area stimulation using stretching, palpation and other corrective techniques may all be used to initiate the movement of Ki in the meridians. These

I

pressure and stretching techniques encourage self-healing, rebalance the body and ease both mental and physical tension.

The History and Philosophy

Historically, Western medical philosophy and application are well documented. From the time of the Father of Medicine, Hippocrates, guidelines were set down for the treatment of disease which were not dissimilar to the treatment principles of Traditional Chinese Medicine. The use of natural remedies including diet, herbalism and massage were all promoted.

The *Nei Ching* (Book of the Interior) is the first recorded medical text of Chinese Medicine. It was written in around 100 BC and is a compilation of material by Huang Ti, the Yellow Emperor. The development of different therapies such as acupuncture, Chinese herbalism, moxibustion (the burning of the mugwart herb on or near the skin) and 'Amma' (Chinese massage) was generally determined by geographic and cultural considerations. In the southern and eastern regions of China acupuncture was common. In the agricultural west the availability of herbs made herbalism popular. In the cold, northern mountainous regions moxibustion was most effective to drive out Cold disorders (*see* page 82). In the more central regions health problems were treated with Amma and corrective exercises.

There has been a long historical relationship between China and Japan. Travel, trade, cross-cultural marriages and war have all contributed to Japanese culture embracing Traditional Chinese Medicine and further developing the same to suit the Japanese people. Japanese massage, called 'Anma', has been used for centuries to deal with many common ailments, from aches and pains to the treatment of more serious illnesses. However, although the basis of shiatsu therapy has grown out of thousands of years of Chinese medicinal principles, it was not until this century that Tokujiro Namikoshi, the initiator of the first style of shiatsu as we know it today, combined the diagnostic and treatment philosophy of acupuncture to create this powerful healing art.

Shiatsu in Japan is quite different from the styles of shiatsu applied here in the West. This is mainly due to cultural attitudes to healing. Shiatsu in Japan tends to be more 'physical' and many deep tissue and manipulative techniques are used, combined with strong stretches. A Westerner would usually find this form of treatment too painful to accept. Because of the strong belief in 'face' in Japan, the average receiver of shiatsu will not express emotional and psychological problems to the practitioner, and the treatment is based at the physical level and physical contact will be strong.

Emotional problems are supposed to be dealt with in private with the family. Here in the West, however, we love to reveal our deepest secrets and have them interpreted and hopefully treated as part of any therapy. Shiatsu is about *living your potential* and opening your mind to the possibilities available to you.

> In the beginner's mind there are many possibilities,
> but in the expert's there are few.
>
> *Shunryu Suzuki*[1]

There are several principal 'styles' of shiatsu found in the West: for example, Barefoot Shiatsu, Macrobiotic Shiatsu, Namikoshi style, Ohashiatsu®, Shiatsu-Do™, Zen Shiatsu, Healing-Shiatsu and Movement Shiatsu. These are all valid and effective therapies using the basic shiatsu principles, but with differing emphasis placed on techniques or philosophy. In Japan there is a distinction between shiatsu massage, a relaxing and invigorating massage technique, and shiatsu therapy, used to treat more serious disorders.

There are more than 87,000 registered shiatsu practitioners in Japan today. This fact alone, we feel, goes some way towards demonstrating the effectiveness of this therapy in the prevention and treatment of disease. Shiatsu is offered to Japanese workers in major industry free of charge as a healthcare method, and most Japanese families will know and use simple shiatsu massage techniques in the home.

How Shiatsu Relates to Women

Women particularly seem to be attracted to shiatsu. Many more women than men come for treatments and the majority of those studying shiatsu as a career are also women. We think that this may be because women tend to be more aware of their own bodies and the concept of feeling good about themselves, whereas men perhaps are more inclined to ignore signs and symptoms of imbalance until much later.

Having a regular (and hard to ignore) body clock in the form of the menstrual cycle also gives women the advantage of obvious signs of imbalance when unexplained changes occur. Let's consider this an advantage and this same indication of imbalance can reveal improvements as your health changes for the better.

Of course men also have various disorders specifically related to their reproductive system physiology and organs, and shiatsu and the general exercises and lifestyle suggestions in this book will benefit them equally.

The psycho-emotional considerations explained come from many of the same fundamental patterns relating to self-image and self-worth, although there are of course psycho-emotional features specific to women, as there are to men. This is the nature of our lives.

How Shiatsu Was Traditionally Used by Japanese Women

Women in both Japanese and Chinese societies historically used shiatsu and massage-type therapies (then known as 'Anma' and 'Amma' respectively), as well as herbal remedies, for the treatment of common ailments.

As an example of how shiatsu treatment has changed over the years, in Japan today and in contemporary Western styles of shiatsu there are a number of contraindicated pressure points which we do not use in the early stages of pregnancy, because of a possible risk of miscarriage. In traditional Oriental societies, however, pregnant women would actively stimulate these same pressure points, as a method of ensuring that only strong children would be born. If the women then miscarried, it was considered a positive event and a sign that they needed to improve their health before again becoming pregnant. They believed that if the spirit of the child was strong and determined, then these very same 'contraindicated' points would enhance a healthier pregnancy.

Understanding the Fundamentals of Shiatsu
Your Life 'Potential'

Life is not a mystery.
It is an art we have
not fully uncarved yet.

Anon.

It may be difficult to come up with a scientific definition for *life,* or even to define it in philosophical terms, but it is quite easy to find characteristics common to all forms of life. First of all, living things never exist until they are born, and when they die they cease to exist. 'Life' is always limited in space and time and its existence totally dependent on the presence of other life.

We came into being through multiple cell division. At the time of conception, one single cell starts to divide and forms billions of cells to develop into a human being. All these billions of cells work together to form a complete unit and to exist as a whole. Surrounding all these billions of cells is a membranous border separating our internal environment from our external environment. As human beings, we use this border for our physical and emotional protection and also communicate across it with others and our external environment.

Although we all exist as individuals, we all depend on other individuals for our survival. To sustain life, there needs to be an exchange of *basic life energy* or *Ki* between individuals.

Your Life Force – The Ki

Essentially, we all have a 'Life Force' or energy which created the physical structure and regulates the physical, emotional, mental and spiritual stability. Your body is your current 'vessel' for the physical manifestation of your Spirit (*see* fig. 1.1). This Life Force (called *Ki* in Japanese and *Qi* or *Chi* in Chinese) maintains a homeostatic balance in your body (internal environment balance). When the Ki is disturbed through external trauma, such as an injury, or internal trauma, such as anxiety and stress, symptoms occur. The shiatsu therapist assesses the distribution of Ki throughout the body and corrects the imbalance accordingly.

fig. 1.1 Energy creates the structure which 'houses' the Mind

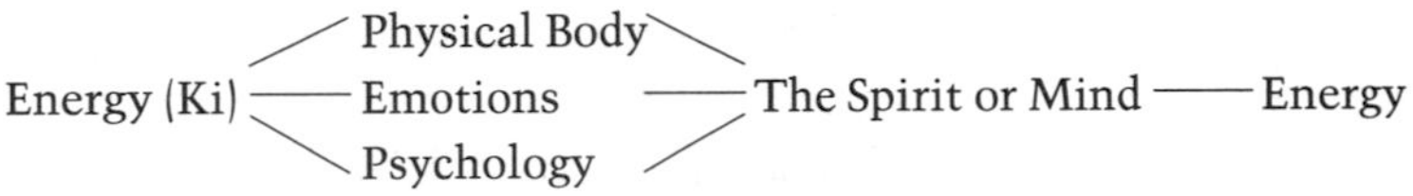

Energy (Ki) — Physical Body / Emotions / Psychology — The Spirit or Mind — Energy

The concept of Ki might be a bit difficult for you to grasp at first, but the idea is fundamental to Oriental medical thinking. The word 'Ki' comes from the original Chinese concept of *Chi* or *Qi*, introduced to the West through acupuncture and the Chinese martial art of t'ai chi ch'uan. The Chinese word *Qi* translates as 'breaths'. If you look in a Japanese dictionary, it defines *Ki* as 'mind, spirit or heart' and lists hundreds of expresions that use the word *Ki* (most of them ordinary ways of talking about human moods, attitudes or character). For example, the Japanese word for describing sickness is *byoki*, which translates as 'troubled Ki'; *genki* means 'source of Ki' or 'health'.

Ki is the 'information' your body needs for maintaining balance. *Information* refers to the communication between the individual body systems to act as an integrated 'whole'. It is much easier to demonstrate Ki than to try to measure or contain it, and there are a variety of exercises you can do to get in touch with Ki and feel the effect of Ki upon your body (*see* the

Do-In exercises in Chapter 7). Ki is a real force, made up of electric, magnetic, infrasonic and infrared vibrations, which can be intuitively perceived and mentally directed. Like the air we breathe and depend on for our life, and the water we take into our bodies, Ki is the very source of our vitality which keeps us alive and living. It is the force within us which gives us initiative, which drives and inspires us to move forwards in life. In Oriental Medicine Ki is considered as our Life *Force* or Life *Essence*, which maintains and nurtures our physical body and therefore also affects our mind and spirit. The human body cannot be separated into individual parts functioning separately from one another: your physical body is a field of continually moving energy, circulating through the cells, muscles and organs.

Ki is everywhere. It moves and changes quickly from moment to moment and it can easily be replenished on a day-to-day basis. As soon as we are born, we start to eat, drink and breathe. Already at this point in life our Lungs, Stomach and Spleen start functioning to produce Ki from food, drink and air and provide us with the 'fuel' we need for our daily activities. Ki is essential for us as living beings and, when the Ki leaves us, we die.

Essence or Jing   Chinese Medicine sees the working of the body and mind as a result of the interaction of certain vital substances called *Fundamental Substances*. These substances manifest themselves in varying degrees, ranging from completely material, such as Body Fluids, to more immaterial, such as Ki described earlier. There is another Fundamental Substance which plays a very important part in our growth and development and that is *Jing* or *Essence*, as it is usually translated. Essence is a precious substance which is inherited from our parents and also partly replenished from the Ki extracted from food. This organic substance which forms the basis for growth, reproduction and development is stored in the Kidneys. It controls our sexual maturation and reproductive function, as well as forming the basis for successful conception and pregnancy. Whereas Ki is the ability to activate and move, Essence is thought of as a more dense form of energy than Ki. Ki is a lighter vibration, Essence is a more pure, almost liquefied substance of high potency (comparable to the potencies of aromatherapy essential oils).

According to the first chapter of the *Simple Questions* women's Essence flows in seven-year cycles:

The Kidney energy of a girl becomes abundant at the age of seven, her baby teeth are replaced by permanent ones and the hair grows.

At the age of 14, the Dew of Heaven arrives (menstruation), the Directing Vessel begins to flow, the Penetrating Vessel is flourishing, the periods come regularly and she can conceive. At the age of 21, the Kidney Essence peaks, the wisdom teeth come out and growth is at its outmost. At the age of 28, tendons and bones become strong, the hair grows longest and the body is strong and flourishing. At the age of 35, the Bright Yang channels begin to weaken, the complexion starts to wither and the hair begins to fall. At the age of 42, the three Yang channels are weak, the face darkens and the hair begins to turn grey. At the age of 49, the Directing Vessel is empty, the Penetrating Vessel depleted, the Dew of Heaven dries up, the Earth Passage [uterus] is not open, so weakness and infertility set in.[2]

The Production of Ki

We produce Ki through the intake and processing of air, food and drink. Combine these substances with the Kidney Essence mentioned earlier and you have your Ki (energy) source. The Kidney Essence acts as the catalyst to begin a percolation process of the Air meeting with the Earth Essences (food and drink). This percolation sends a bubbling of energy throughout your whole system which mixes with the inherent energies of each organ to establish a homeostatic balance of Ki. Ki has six basic functions: warming, transporting, transforming, supporting, raising and protecting your organ Ki (the Ki produced, stored, distributed and used by your internal organs) in your internal environment.

Yin/Yang and You

Eastern philosophy is based on the concept that human beings are an integral part of the universe. In the same way that trees, clouds and animals are all subject to the law of nature, so, too, are we as human beings. If you live according to the law of nature and adapt to the different changing cycles, the quality of your Ki will be maintained and you will be healthy and productive. It is when you fail to adapt that you are more likely to become ill.

The Oriental medical system follows a fundamental principle – that is, everything is affected by and is part of a phenomenon of nature known as *Yin* and *Yang*. Yin/Yang theory maintains that all things are essentially composed of these two opposing, yet complementary aspects, and that all phenomena naturally group themselves into complementary pairs of opposites. Nothing is solely Yin or Yang; everything is composed of both in varying degrees. Nothing is neutral; either Yin or Yang predominates. This is the process of change. Everything in nature changes all the time, nothing is completely still: day turns to night and back to day again; the seasons move in a continuous cycle of change; we as human beings are born, live our lives and then die. Everything has a cycle.

If all things are affected by Yin and Yang, so are you as a human being and a woman. Yang is thought of as being the more male or masculine force, Yin the more female force. But as stated earlier, everything is composed of both in varying degrees. Oriental philosophy describes Yin as 'shade' (cooling) and Yang as 'sunlight' (heating). The shade is an analogy for the night and the Moon, the sunlight for daylight and the Sun influence.

Different parts of your body are more Yang, other parts of your body have a more Yin quality. The upper part of your body, the back and your skin (your outer surface) are considered to be more Yang areas; your lower body, your abdomen and bones (deeper in your body) are more Yin. In general, we can say that areas higher up and more to the surface are more Yang, whereas the interior and lower parts of your body are more Yin. We also think of Yin as more soft and open in quality (your abdomen), Yang as more hard and protective (your back).

Yin is the 'Water' nature of your body. This refers to the cooling function of Yin, as well as its storage tendency. Yin is stored in the organs and also in the joints and muscle tendons. Yang is the 'Fire' nature of the body – that is, its heating function, as well as the process of activating the stored Ki into movement needed for your life. Ki is synonymous with movement and is agitated if 'held'.

When it comes to your internal organs and reproductive system, a woman's reproductive organs are thought of as being influenced predominately by Yin energy, as they are located deeper in the body and have a more dense structure, especially the primary organs, the ovaries. A man's primary organs of reproduction have more of a Yang influence and are located externally, especially the primary organs of the testes, which also have a less dense structure.

The Energy System

Ki circulates throughout your body along specific pathways or channels of energy known as *meridians.* Meridians act like an efficient irrigation system, ensuring the nurturing of all bodily functions when energy is flowing without disturbance. There are 12 major meridians and 5 *Extraordinary Vessels* (further discussed in Chapter 5) used in shiatsu (*see* figs 1.2–1.17), each supplying energy to a specific internal organ or system. The Extraordinary Vessels control and regulate the 12 major meridians. The meridians are named according to the internal organ they effect and are bilateral – that is, there is an identical meridian on both sides of your body. The meridians connect all different body parts with each other and ensure proper nurturing of Ki throughout your whole being. When you are healthy, the flow of Ki proceeds unlocked and energy is well distributed throughout the meridian pathways.

The 12 meridian/organ functions are divided into six pairs – that is, six Yin and six Yang meridian/organ functions:

Yin	**Yang**
Lung (LU)	Large Intestine (LI)
Spleen (SP)	Stomach (ST)
Heart (HT)	Small Intestine (SI)
Kidney (KID)	Bladder (BL)
Heart Governor (HG)	Triple Burner (TB)
Liver (LIV)	Gall Bladder (GB)

Should a meridian become blocked, the area or internal organ/system connected to this meridian will then enter a state of *dis-ease* or a condition of stress. Dis-ease is a sign that the energy within the meridian is out of balance. Along the meridians you will find more highly charged energy points, which we call pressure points or *tsubo* in Japanese. This is where the Ki is most easily affected and we will teach you later on in the book how to apply pressure onto these different points, in order to change and rebalance your Ki within. All pressure points are numbered showing their location – for example, LIV 3, the third point on the Liver meridian. They also have specific names relating to their function (although we will not refer to these so often).

When we talk about the energy (Ki) of an organ of the meridian system, we refer to its energy 'storage and production' function or its 'activating' function in terms of it being in a state of Ki *Deficiency* (lacking vitality) or Ki *Excess* (too much vitality). Both these conditions may cause signs of disharmony. These are signs of Ki stagnation – that is, the Ki is not flowing in the organ and meridian in a 'free-flowing' and uninhibited manner, necessary for maintaining the health of an organism. For good health, you need the proper production and storage of your Ki, combined with the effective utilization of that Ki into movement.

To describe this in another way, imagine a locked grain storehouse filled to capacity and surrounded by a starving populace who do not have the key for the storehouse door. The grain is the Yin (stored energy), and the door key would be the Yang, the 'activity' function needed to release the Yin. This would be a Ki Excess condition.

When we use the term 'Spleen Ki', for example, we are referring to the function of the Stomach meridian and organ in terms of its efficiency in relation to the other organ/meridians or a body tissue such as the 'flesh' (muscles). This is an expression of its health and vitality or disharmony. For example, 'rebellious Stomach Ki' is a term describing an upwards movement of energy manifesting as vomiting.

Each organ also has a Yin function and a Yang function. For example, Liver Yin is the Liver's ability to store Ki and Blood. As in the example of the grain storehouse above, without the Liver Yang (activating) function, this stored Ki and Blood cannot be utilized by your body. The Yang function of the organ/meridians also refers to their emotional expressions which are intangible and are not dense like the organs themselves. Angry outbursts, therefore, are another example of your Liver Yang.

By using different shiatsu techniques, such as pressure, stretching, rubbing and corrective exercises, you will soon be able to release the blockages, 'open' the meridian and recharge yourself.

fig. 1.2 (top)
Lung meridian
(LU) *Metal (Yin)*

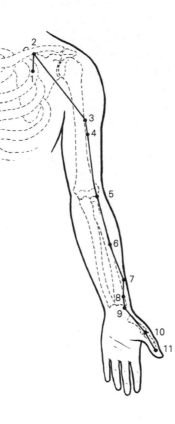

fig. 1.3 (right)
Large Intestine meridian
(LI) *Metal (Yang)*

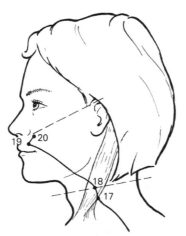

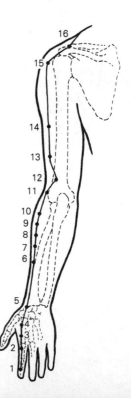

fig. 1.4
Stomach meridian
(ST) *Earth (Yang)*

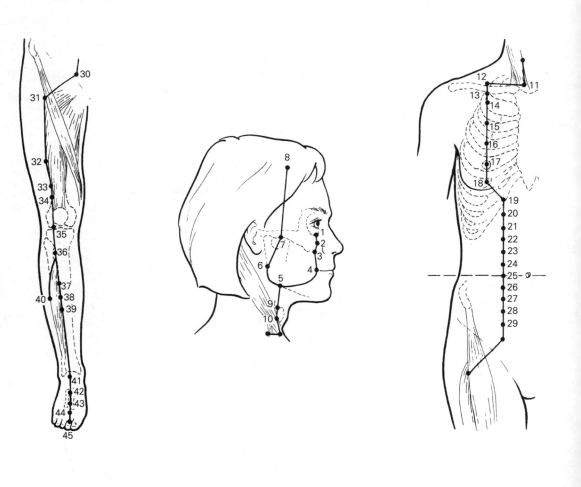

fig. 1.5 Spleen meridian
(SP) *Earth (Yin)*

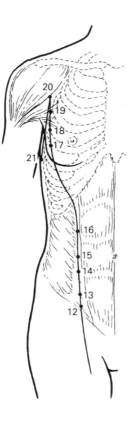
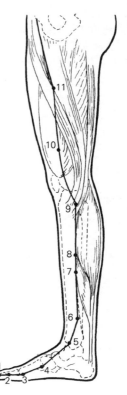

fig. 1.6 Heart meridian
(HT) *Fire (Yin)*

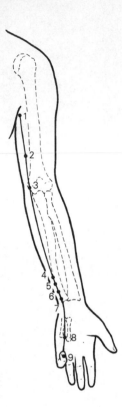

fig. 1.7 Small Intestine
meridian
(SI) *Fire (Yang)*

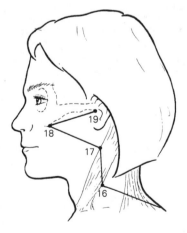

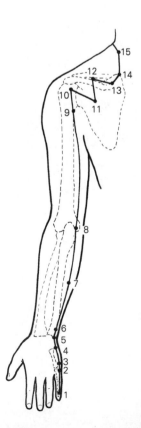

fig. 1.8 Bladder meridian
(BL) *Water (Yang)*

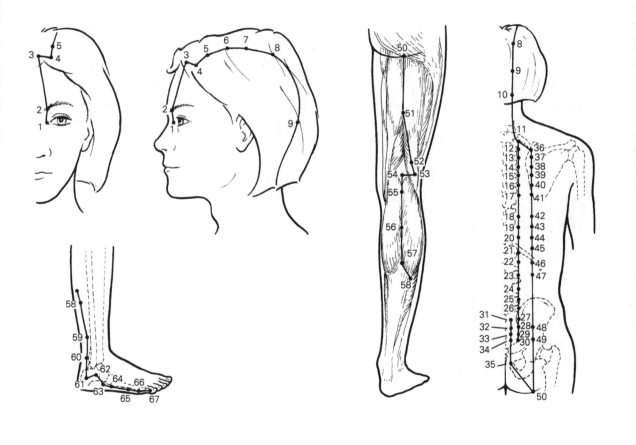

fig. 1.9 (right)
Kidney meridian
(KID) *Water (Yin)*

fig. 1.10 (below) Heart
Governor meridian
(HG) *Fire (Yin)*

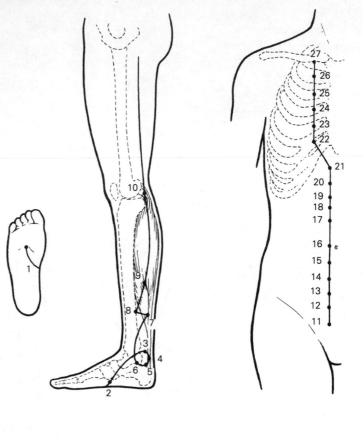

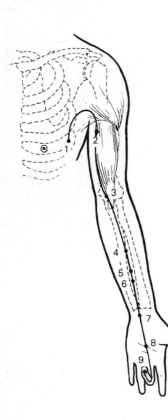

fig. 1.11 (below right)
Triple Burner meridian
(TB) *Fire (Yang)*

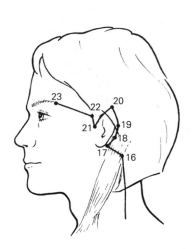

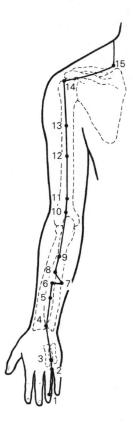

fig. 1.12
Gall Bladder meridian
(GB) *Wood (Yang)*

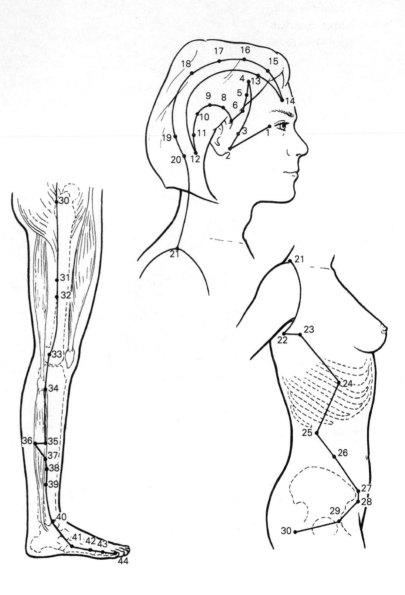

fig. 1.13
Liver meridian
(LIV) *Wood (Yin)*

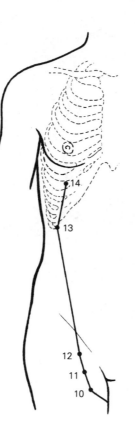

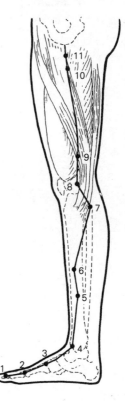

fig. 1.14
Conception Vessel
(Ren Mai)
(cv)

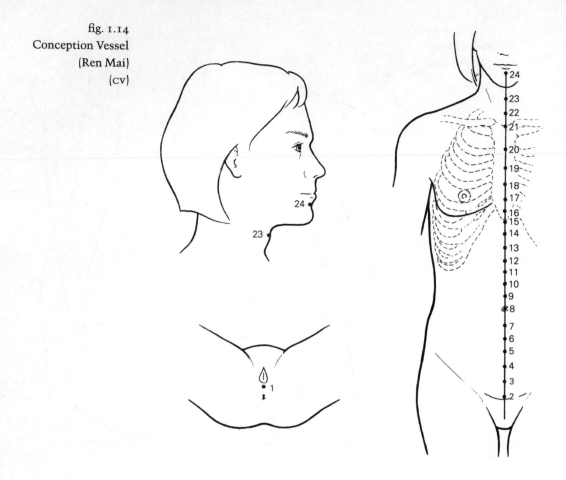

fig. 1.15
Governing Vessel
(Du Mai)
(GV)

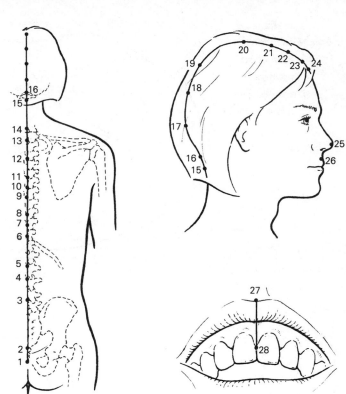

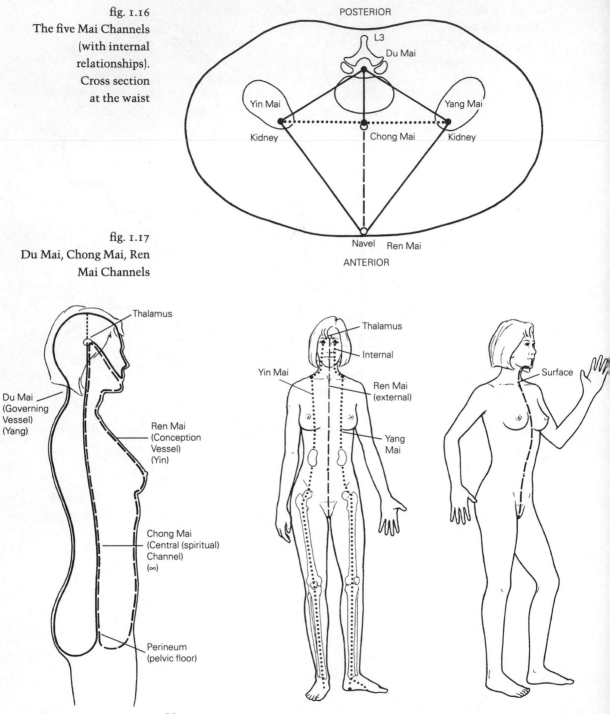

fig. 1.16
The five Mai Channels
(with internal
relationships).
Cross section
at the waist

POSTERIOR

L3
Du Mai

Yin Mai   Yang Mai

Kidney   Chong Mai   Kidney

Navel   Ren Mai

ANTERIOR

fig. 1.17
Du Mai, Chong Mai, Ren
Mai Channels

Thalamus

Du Mai
(Governing
Vessel)
(Yang)

Ren Mai
(Conception
Vessel)
(Yin)

Chong Mai
(Central (spiritual)
Channel)
(∞)

Perineum
(pelvic floor)

Thalamus

Internal

Yin Mai

Ren Mai
(external)

Yang
Mai

Surface

22

Left (Yang) Mai and right (Yin) Mai

The Breath of Life –
Air as Energy

A fundamental process of Life is respiration. All animals need oxygen to sustain them, and the quality and quantity of oxygen consumed have a direct effect on vitality and stamina. The energy received in respiration is called 'Air Ki', and this Ki is transformed by the Lungs into a usable form.

There are both external and internal causes which may upset the Lung Ki. Polluted air, smoking, air conditioning and poor diet (especially dairy products) will all adversely affect your breathing potential. The incidence of adult and childhood asthma is dramatically increasing in today's society, mainly due to these external causes. The internal causes relate to your emotions. Grief, sadness and depression all reside in the chest and affect your *Shen* (translated as 'spirit' or 'mind'), which in turn affects your posture, which then affects your physical organ structures. A vicious circle is created. Sayings such as 'Get it off your chest' and 'Spit it out' when alluding to repressed emotions are referring to stagnant Chest Ki and, therefore, Lung Ki.

The breathing reflex is stimulated in the base of the brain (the *medulla oblongata)* which sends motor messages to the lungs to become active. The lungs then take in air and refresh your blood by oxygenating it. This oxygenated (Ki-charged) blood is pumped to the brain, which is the largest consumer of blood in the body, and provides the vitality for your motor and sensory nerve functions. The better the quality of this blood, the better nervous system responses. So, when you don't breathe well (that is, shallow and quick) or take in polluted air, the poor quality blood will feed your brain and lessen your body potential. Poor breathing equals poor brain activity, equals poor organ activity – so breathe deep and wake up your brain.

Food Is your Fuel –
The Fire in your Blood

The other main source of Ki intake is through food. Whereas the lungs take in the air, the stomach takes in food and drink. In a process referred to as 'rotting and ripening', the churning processes of the stomach allow the breakdown of food and drink. This food source is converted into an Essence by the Spleen, which acts as a building block for the creation of Blood and is referred to as the 'Nutritive Ki'. Blood has a different meaning .from the Western view of the red liquid substance in your veins and refers to purified Ki. The Essence filters to the Lung, where it mixes with the Lung Mist and is 'fired' by the Yang of the Heart. The Heart in turn activates these substances which form the Blood for circulation throughout your body. The Chinese saw this latter process as the Heart 'stamping the red of fire' on the Blood.

Poor diet creates poor Blood quality and, since Blood is a Fundamental Substance of the body, the body's activities (including the functions of the reproductive organs) will be diminished. Poor diet is greatly responsible for disorders such as diabetes, asthma, heart disease, skin problems and digestive and reproductive complaints. The Spleen is most affected and this influences your self-image and sense of security. Imbalances of the Spleen might manifest themselves as strong sweet cravings, a loss of self-confidence, poor lymph flow, the loss of muscle tonus, sagging and/or 'pitted' flesh, feeling cynical about things or a need to be 'mothered' and not 'smothered'.

chapter 2

What Shiatsu Can Do for You

How Shiatsu Helps

It is easy to learn the basics of shiatsu because it is so enjoyable and definitely has a 'feel good' factor. The 'taking care of yourself' aspect is also very important, as it acknowledges your value as a person and empowers you to create change where necessary. The combination of self-treatment techniques, stretch exercises and Do-In exercises (*see* Chapter 7) will help you to improve both physically and mentally. Some simple responses will be the relief of joint or muscle stiffness, increased mobility and flexibility, strengthened bones, improved immunity, greater elimination of toxins and the alleviation of fatigue.

The effects may be physical, emotional or both. Shiatsu also affects the way you think, not just about yourself, but about life in general. It often brings out the more philosophical attributes in a woman. Shiatsu treats your well-being and the symptoms of this affect different women in differing ways. The energy system is our primary concern and is given greater importance than physiological considerations. The physiology of shiatsu is Yin and Yang, which are not Western models, but this does not mean that the reactions will not be physically or emotionally discernible.

Shiatsu can help women to:

- relieve stress
- strengthen the body, mind and spirit
- improve general health and well-being
- enhance skin tone by stimulating and revitalizing the skin
- improve muscle flexibility
- improve posture
- calm the nervous system
- improve digestion
- stimulate blood and lymph circulation
- achieve emotional and psychological balance
- alleviate premenstrual tension
- slow the ageing process
- make the hair more vital
- increase stamina
- enhance libido and sexual enjoyment
- promote healthy pregnancy and aid childbirth
- relieve aches and pains, back and neck ache
- prevent common illnesses
- more accurately interpret the rhythms of the body and create greater body awareness

Emotional and Psychological Benefits

Stiff and tight muscles, aching with fatigue? Shoulders slowly embracing your ears as those neck muscles seize up? Yes, this is tension caused by stress. By learning how to improve your physical posture in everyday situations – such as sitting, standing, working and sleeping – you can dramatically reduce tension. By learning to improve your 'emotional posture', you can influence your response to stress levels and thus reduce the physical reactions. You will learn these skills with shiatsu.

Does your abdomen knot up and do your bowels scream when you are stressed? Do your shoulders collapse and your back ache when you feel depressed? These are all physical reactions to emotional stress, which can be controlled both by your mind and by moving your body. Remember, every woman is subjected to stress every day: noise and air pollution, traffic congestion, family frictions, to name but a few. The determining factor between you and the next person is how you *react* to these everyday stresses. Empower yourself with the choice: 'Will I get stressed about this or not?'

By asking yourself this question, you put yourself in 'control'. Stress feels like an attack (usually termed 'anxiety attack') precisely because you have lost control.

In shiatsu, we do not distinguish between mind and body as separate entities. Stress that affects the mind will create physical symptoms, and physical stress will result in psychological symptoms. Seeking help from a therapy which (unlike shiatsu) only deals with the mind, or only with physical disharmonies, does not consider the inseparable relationship of the bodymind.

Mood swings from day to day are not unusual, and your moods are influenced by many factors, including the weather, your work, family relationships and your moon cycle. It is when you feel stuck in a pattern of emotional expression, or lack of expression, that these 'patterns' become fixed. At this stage we think of them as psychological patterns – that is, more deeply rooted and fixed, causing you to react in certain ways. Your mood swings are signs of stagnant Ki. Shiatsu will help free this stagnation by releasing deeper 'held' emotions and traumas from your past.

In this book we regularly refer to your 'potential' being inhibited or released. *Potential* here refers to your appetite for enjoying your life and the realization of your dreams or destiny. Are you happy in your relationship or work life? Do you feel in a rut, unable to take control of your direction and happiness? These are inhibitions to your potential being realized. You have a choice – that is, either to give yourself empowerment in what you wish to achieve in your life or to be disempowered, firstly by yourself, and then by others. Many people feel that this is one of the greatest benefits of shiatsu – the sighting of your self-empowerment.

The Physical Benefits
Revitalizing your Skin
Your skin has a breathing capacity and also acts as a physical layer of protection against the invasion of pathogens (external environmental influences – dampness, cold, heat, wind and dryness). Both these functions come under the control of the *Defensive Ki* of the body called *Wei Ki*. This is referred to as being 'fierce and courageous' and protects you on both an emotional and physical level. The Wei Ki is controlled by your Lung function and regulates the opening and closing of the skin pores. Your ability to effectively detoxify and eliminate waste (the 'impure' energy left over after processing your air and food intake) is reflected in your skin condition.

Shiatsu will enhance the quality of your Lung Ki, thus eliminating toxins more effectively, leaving your skin glowing and you feeling more positive.

Toning your Muscular System

Your muscles give you the ability to move. Their main functions are locomotion, protection and heat manufacture. Your 'direction' in life is also aided by the freedom of movement of the muscles. Stiff and tense muscles may reflect a stiff and tense approach to the hurdles in your life and act as mirrors for the flexibility of your thinking and emotions.

The muscular system comes under the control of the Liver and Spleen functions. The Liver Ki nourishes the stabilizing structures of a joint – the ligaments, tendons and cartilage. Weakened joints are generally a sign of Liver Deficiency and may be caused by overuse of a joint or the intake of foods which may weaken the tissue, such as an excess of refined sugars or alcohol.

The Spleen Ki regulates the tone, elasticity and lubrication of the 'flesh' or muscle body. When the Spleen is weakened, the muscles will tend to sag. This is commonly more apparent in women than men.

Because shiatsu is working directly on the skin surface and penetrates to the muscle tissue, the muscles respond to the touch by relaxing. Stimulating the Spleen and Liver meridians will create a better flow of Blood, Ki and lymph and ensure better nourishment of the muscles.

Strengthening your Skeletal System

Protection and support are the primary functions of the skeletal system in Western thinking. The bones contain marrow which, physiologically, is involved in blood production. The Oriental concept of the Marrow is different. It is created out of Essence, a pure form of liquefied energy stored in the Kidneys. The *Pre-Heaven Essence* – the foundations of human development created at the time of conception from the meeting of parental ovum and sperm (Yin and Yang energies respectively) – provides the strength of your constitution during embryonic development. The *Post-Heaven Essence* is contributed by the proper dietary and environmental influences of early infancy, up to about the age of two. The combination of the Pre- and Post-Heaven Essence is referred to as *Jing* (your constitutional vitality and strength). The health of your parents at your conception, together with the subsequent embryonic phase and infancy, all help to determine your constitutional strengths or weaknesses.

In Oriental thought, therefore, this Marrow is the basis for the creation of the physiological bone marrow and forms the foundation for the structure of the brain and spinal cord. We can thus say that the contin-ued health of the brain and spinal cord, which form your central nervous system, is maintained by the Kidney Ki.

The Kidney Ki also regulates bone health and maintenance (including your teeth), hearing and head hair, as well as the residence of the Jing. The physical manifestation of Jing in a woman is the ovum, in a man, the sperm. During the natural ageing process, the Jing is depleted and so ageing occurs. The bones become 'dry' as the potency of the marrow is exhausted; the teeth degenerate; head hair is lost or becomes grey (another indication of the 'drying' of the Essence); brain vitality is reduced and comprehension and concentration become limited. If all or some of these symptoms are happening prematurely, the individual concerned is living a lifestyle that is prematurely exhausting the Jing. This is very common due to excess work, stress, sex or alcohol, drug abuse or multiple childbirths.

Shiatsu will help to slow down the Kidney Jing depletion and, there-fore, maintain healthier bones by tonifying the Kidney Ki. Attention to a more regulated life routine – balancing work and leisure with exercise and good diet – will also improve the Kidney strength.

Stimulating your Circulatory System
The heart organ and the Heart and Heart Governor Ki are the central focus for circulation regulation and maintenance of the blood. The Spleen Ki 'holds the blood in place' – that is, prevents it moving recklessly, such as in internal bleeding conditions or bleeding outside of a woman's ordinary menstruation. The lymph – responsible for waste removal via the blood and lymph nodes – is transported and regulated by the Spleen and Triple Burner functions.

The condition of the heart and Heart Ki (Fire energy) is weakened dra-matically by poor diet and lack of exercise. External influences, such as excess Heat, will injure the functioning of the Heart Ki, and lead to heat rising in the body, congestion of the chest and head, thus leaving the pelvis and extremities depleted. This usually occurs in overly heated houses and during long exposure to the sun or other heat sources. Regular exposure to Heat may also cause a drying of the body fluids.

There is also the internal Heat of anger, passion or sadness which can injure the Heart Ki. The Heart is the residence of your *Shen* or Spirit. Shen is also sometimes translated as the 'Mind' and refers to your state of well-being. Anger – regulated by the Liver – builds up a heat when repressed, which eventually rises to the chest to injure the Heart. An example of this is a heart attack brought on by an angry outburst. The heat of passion can nurture or injure the Heart Ki, depending on its intensity and direction. Sadness depletes the Heart Ki and 'disturbs the Shen'. All of these conditions may lead to poor sleep patterns, erratic body temperature changes, disturbed concentration, nervous stress, hypertension, mood swings and a generally agitated nature. Shiatsu will help to calm the Shen and thus prevent these problems.

Calming your Nervous System

Your nervous system, divided into two different functional parts – the 'conscious' or somatic nervous system and the 'unconscious' or autonomic nervous system – is regulated by the Kidney and Bladder Ki. The somatic nervous system controls body functions, from the muscle movement of the muscular skeletal system to the excretion of wastes via urination and defecation. Incontinence is therefore partially due to loss of 'conscious' control of the organ muscles involved. It is also via this system that you receive information about pleasure and pain. Both these responses can be controlled.

Your autonomic nervous system controls body activities such as breathing, digestion, circulation, hormonal regulation and genitourinary functions (blood purification, waste control, ovulation and menstruation, for example). Stress is a huge contributor to the restriction of the effective functioning of this part of your nervous system. The autonomic nervous system also controls the 'fight or flight' mechanism, activated in stress situations to prevent injury. This response is provided by a reaction in the adrenal glands, controlled by the Kidney Ki. Adrenal stimulation is activated by danger, visual excitement such as an exciting movie or book (your body becomes tense in expectation), sexual excitement and ingested stimulants such as caffeine, nicotine and some recreational drugs.

Small amounts of adrenal stimulation are not harmful, but in our society many people live in a pressurized and hyper-adrenal state, overly stressed and ready for reaction to danger. This leads to a lack of 'peace' and the constant search for further sustained mental stimulation to prevent boredom. Balancing the energy in the Kidney and Bladder channels through shiatsu will have a calming effect on the nervous system and create a 'switch' from the sympathetic nervous system being in charge to the parasympathetic nervous system, thus calming down all internal activities.

Activating your Digestive System

Your digestive system is responsible for the ingestion and digestion of food and drink. The transformation of the 'pure' from the 'impure', and subsequent transportation of these for absorption and excretion, is regulated by the Stomach and Spleen Ki. 'We are what we eat' is a well-used phrase, but it is as true as it ever was. Food is the foundation for the creation of your Blood. This is the energy source for body maintenance and growth. For example, as a woman, if you do not nurture yourself properly through food and drink, your body could enter a state of Blood Deficiency (lack of Blood). This might manifest itself as reduced or no blood flow. For this reason, it is not recommended to do any prolonged fasting. You can read more about the creation of Blood in Chapter 10.

Food and drink are churned in the stomach and allowed to 'rot and ripen', which creates a purified substance or Essence. Impure substances are further processed and absorbed, or excreted via urination and defecation. When you overeat or chew quickly and too little, you burden your digestive system. For you to achieve the maximum potential from food, you need to consider the food quality, digestion, absorption – this starts with saliva production created by regular chewing of at least 50 times per mouthful – and excretion. If you are constipated, this will usually mean Dryness (Yin Deficiency) and, conversely, excess Damp will create loose bowels.

Another feature of digestion is the intake and transformation of 'information'. A 'hunger' for knowledge might lead to mental fatigue and single-mindedness in its pursuit, leaving the Stomach in a state of Excess. Sedating the energy in the Stomach channel through shiatsu will bring this Excess to a more balanced state and prevent symptoms such as indigestion, constipation, colitis and diverticulitis conditions.

We also live in a society that promotes a strong hunger or greed for material possessions and status. This particular 'hunger' in itself is a stress factor, and when material goals are not achieved, we see ourselves as failures. Surplus leads to stagnation, just as overeating leads to weight gain, which is an unnecessary burden for your body/mind. The Buddhists say that there are two significant times that lead to stress: the stress of wanting to achieve your goals, and the disappointment of actually achieving them.

Balancing your Endocrine (Hormonal) System

Your endocrine system is responsible for the regulation of all glands and tissues that produce hormones. Your bodily activities are regulated through the secretion of hormones, which are transported by the blood via your cardiovascular system. Combined with your nervous system, it coordinates the functions of all your body systems. The hormones are chemical messengers in your bloodstream. Since your blood travels to all body tissues, the hormonal influence is fundamental to homeostasis – that is, the ability of your 'internal' environment to remain within certain physiological limits, particularly when subjected to changes in the 'external' environment.

The endocrine system is made up of ductless glands, of which the 'executive' is the pituitary gland. The other endocrine glands are the thyroid, parathyroids, adrenals, pineal and thymus. In addition to these, there are some organs in you body which contain endocrine tissue, but are not exclusively endocrine glands. In the female body, these are the hypothalamus, pancreas, ovaries, kidneys, stomach and small intestine. The placenta formed in pregnancy also contains endocrine tissue.

Other glands in your body are known as 'exocrine glands', and these are ducted glands (glands that secrete substances through a duct onto the inner surface of an organ or the outer surface of the body). These are responsible for the secretion regulation of body fluids, such as sweat and the skin-lubricating oils of the sebaceous tissue. Your internal mucus production and digestive glands are influenced by the exocrine glands.

Your hormonal function, in energetic terms, is regulated by your Kidney Ki. In your brain, sitting about 3–5 centimetres directly behind the point between your eyebrows, is your pituitary gland. It is this gland which, amongst other commanding functions, tells your ovaries to release the hormones needed in menstrual regulation and the ovulation cycle.

The careful maintenance of your Kidney Jing is fundamental to a long and healthy mental and physical life. Your ovaries, and especially the ovum, are the structural 'expression' of the Kidney Jing. Early menopause, when the ovum supply is exhausted, is thus an indication of prematurely exhausted Kidney Jing. Factors which commonly stress the Kidney energy are poor diet, excess work, sex, intake of stimulants including coffee, tobacco and alcohol, and childbirth. Regular shiatsu treatments with tonification and balancing of your Kidney energy will help prevent the premature depletion of your Jing.

Awakening your Lymph and Immune Systems

Your lymph system is responsible for the transportation of proteins and fats via the cardiovascular system. It is also responsible for the filtering of body fluids, the production of white blood cells and immunity control. It comprises lymphatic vessels, structures and organs containing lymphatic tissue. This tissue is made up of large numbers of white blood cells called 'lymphocytes', which are fundamental to the functioning of your immune system. Lymph organ structures include your spleen, thymus gland, lymph nodes appearing throughout your body, and tonsils. Unfortunately, the tonsils are commonly removed in childhood, which actually has the effect of blocking the energy centre in this area, responsible for verbal communication and expression of emotions and thoughts. More frequent upper respiratory tract disorders also become more apparent in these people.

The Spleen function of transforming and transporting energy is the main influence on your lymphatic system. Therefore, signs such as swelling in your armpits, or groin lymph nodes, show Spleen Ki disharmony. Oedema and abdominal bloating show Liver and Kidney Ki stagnation. There is usually some Lung Ki imbalance also presiding, as the Lungs determine the quality of the Ki.

It is a common response to a shiatsu treatment for the receiver to experience elimination reactions which we call 'discharges'. These can be headaches, boils, muscle aches, flu-type symptoms or fatigue. These reactions all serve as indicators that the toxins residing in your body have been activated by your awakened lymphatic system, and are now eliminating via your bloodstream. You need to keep an objective view as these discharges occur, and keep telling yourself that it is cleaning your system and doing you good.

chapter 3

Shiatsu Tools and Techniques

Dos and Don'ts (Contraindications)

Giving shiatsu to yourself or a friend is both relaxing and enjoyable. It can be lots of fun and have a nurturing and healing effect. However, we think it is best to bring in early considerations of what to do and what not to do, to save unnecessary discomfort or stress.

You can give and receive shiatsu as frequently as you wish. It can be used for helping a vast variety of conditions or simply as a method of relaxation or stress management. There are times or circumstances, however, when shiatsu is not appropriate, or when someone should be referred to a professional therapist or medical doctor. The first rule is: *use your common sense.*

You need to consider both your own condition and the condition of your receiver (if you are treating yourself then obviously you count as the receiver as well as the giver). Do *not* give a shiatsu treatment if the receiver:

- has a high fever
- is intoxicated
- has just eaten – wait two hours after meals
- has chronic high blood pressure – seek medical advice
- has a history of brain haemorrhage
- has blood-borne cancer

- is in the first trimester of pregnancy – seek professional advice
- has a skin or air 'contact' contagious disease (HIV/AIDS is of course OK, as no body fluids are exchanged in shiatsu)

Also remember the following if the receiver:

- has had recent surgery – do not apply direct pressure techniques
- has her period – do not apply heavy pressure to the abdomen
- is wearing an intrauterine device (IUD) – do not apply deep pressure to the lower abdomen
- has varicose veins – do not apply pressure directly over the veins

Do *not* give shiatsu if you:

- are too fatigued or are intoxicated
- have a skin or air 'contact' contagious disease
- do not want to give a treatment – ask yourself why!

Giving a Treatment – Making Friends
It is really useful to have a partner for those times when you want to practise your shiatsu techniques or, more often, want someone else to relieve your aches and stress. You can practise techniques by applying pressure to pillows or even the family pet, but it never quite gives the same 'high' as a real, live, human volunteer. If you have or can 'borrow' a young child, get them to walk on the back of your legs, buttocks and back area (avoid walking directly on the spine). This is fun and feels great too. Giving treatments to children is easy, confidence-building and very rewarding. If it is your aching period pains that you want to alleviate, or those of your daughter or friend, you'll find that giving and receiving shiatsu will help you both, mentally and physically.

1 + 1 = 1? From Separation to Unification
Shiatsu is great for building relationships. Two people with entirely different lives and backgrounds can come together for a shiatsu treatment. You, or both of you, are wanting to try out some techniques, experiment really, and think it might be a relaxing experience. You start with separate ideas or expectations as separate individuals. It is your job to 'communicate' to this person your good intentions. You are presumably doing this with some idea of helping them, so it is a two-way communication at least.

Empty Mind or 'Baby' Mind

When you sit quietly beside your partner, just take a few deep breaths and calm your mind. Try to create the state of *Empty Mind* or *'Baby' Mind* – like a baby seeing and feeling a rattle for the first time, their mind free of distractions and all of their 'being' concentrated and focused on this rattle. This mind is 'empty' and so may be filled with new information.

With a hand gently resting on your partner's sacrum (the large wedge-shaped bone in the lower part of the back), you can feel their breathing, body temperature, tension or relaxation. This is called 'tuning into' your partner. Part of achieving the Empty Mind is to let go of your own ego and dissolve ideas of Self. Let your mind be filled with information about your partner – is the breathing regular and deep, is the area you touch warm and well toned, do you feel them relaxing under your touch? When your partner has your total concentration, then you are no longer two separate people – your Ki has touched and you will feel 'in tune' more and more as the treatment progresses. Many people feel they just want to hug each other after a treatment, as a new relationship has been established.

Your Treatment Approach

The first consideration in giving shiatsu is *how* to touch. *Touch* can be relaxing, stimulating or even painful. Different people, different signs and symptoms, require a different treatment approach and differing techniques. Is it going to be a deep tissue-stimulating or a *movement*-style treatment, involving rocking and stretching-style techniques, which will disperse Excess Ki? Or will it be a more *stillness*-style treatment, with many gentler 'holding' techniques, encouraging an already tired and Deficient system to restore itself by gathering in its reserves? This latter method may even include working 'off the body', in the etheric layer of Ki.

Your treatment approach is an important issue but usually common sense will prevail. Would you look at your 90-year-old granny – frail and maybe a little bit nervous of what you are proposing – and think, 'Right, I'll just roll her around the futon for a bit, then rock her until her teeth rattle, followed by a touch of sumo wrestling stretch holds'? This would obviously not be the most appropriate decision and, in fact, would probably do her more harm than good, as you will 'disperse' her already Deficient Ki right out of her. If you are treating an athletic person with good flexibility, whose idea of relaxation is doing 40 press-ups between their breakfast Weetabix and toast, someone who likes 'a good, strong stretch' occasionally, then go ahead with a movement-style treatment. Your average treatment partner will probably be somewhere in between these two examples and require a proportion of both treatment styles. Remember, always *ask* your partner if it feels OK.

Touch and Pressure Application

If, at the end of your treatment, your own impression of your touch could be described as feeling like a supporting and empathetic embrace, then you should be satisfied with yourself. If your partner feels the same about the touch, then all the better. Try to use your hand as an extension of your heart. Let your hand mould to the contours of your partner's muscles and flesh. Practise this by shaking hands with someone; note how your whole hand is moulded to that of your partner. Use this same contact theory in your shiatsu. Your touch needs to be very light for some energy 'listening' techniques, and very firm for deep tissue work. We would not use the word 'hard' to describe any firm pressure, as this has connotations of being sharp and rough.

The 'Switch'

In shiatsu we always allow both hands to be in contact with the receiver. One hand is the 'listening' hand, which is stationary; the other is the 'messenger' hand, the active partner going out to do what the listening hand directs. The balancing of these two hands is the essence of shiatsu. Imagine that you have your hands on a sausage-shaped balloon. When you press with just one hand, this pressure creates a distortion and the balloon swells away from the pressure. This distortion is an imbalance and creates an area of Excess (an area of built-up Ki congestion) and a corresponding 'void' or Deficiency (an area depleted of Ki) (*see* fig. 3.1). As you apply pressure with the first hand (listening hand), start to apply a balancing pressure into your messenger hand, with the intention of creating a balanced pressure between the two. The result of this is that the balloon will not suffer distortion and you will feel an almost equal resistance in both hands (*see* fig. 3.2).

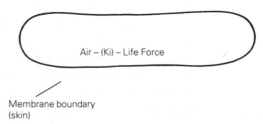

Air – (Ki) – Life Force

Membrane boundary
(skin)

fig. 3.1 Ki in a state of
Excess and Deficiency

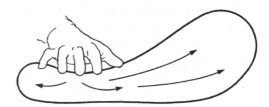

One hand pressure distorts the Ki flow

fig. 3.2 Ki in balance

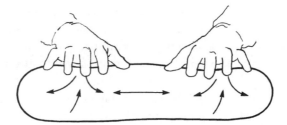

Two hand pressure activates a balancing of Ki

At this point something interesting happens to your autonomic nervous system (ANS) – your 'unconscious' nervous system which controls functions such as breathing and peristalsis (the muscular movement of digestion). It does a 'switch' from being on the defensive (its activating mode), to becoming more passive (its slowing, resting mode). The autonomic nervous system consists of two primary aspects. These are the sympathetic (derived from 'sympathy') and the parasympathetic systems. In very simple terms, the sympathetic system is responsible for gearing you into action (Yang), and the parasympathetic system creates more relaxation and introspection functions (Yin).

When you are touched aggressively, the sympathetic system becomes defensive and creates a tightening and closing of the muscle tissue and organ functions, in preparation for potential pain. The 'fight or flight' mechanism is initiated. Wei Ki (the fierce and courageous defensive energy) is stimulated and becomes Excess. Should the touch be gentle and caring, then your body will initially decipher and interpret these intentions of the touch. Once satisfied of the absence of danger, the sympathetic nervous system steps back and graciously hands over to the parasympathetic system to encourage relaxation and openness. This is when the healing process begins and it is referred to as the *Switch*.

39

The Switch occurs at this point of change between the two systems and this response is felt in the meridian and tsubo you are treating as a pulsation or a softening. Your listening hand usually feels this Switch first and the messenger hand follows. Some people compare this feeling to a flower opening or butter melting. The feeling is one of relief after initial tension. Where there is Excess (*Jitsu* in Japanese), the Switch will be quite rapid, as there is a lot of Ki moving; when the condition is one of Deficiency (*Kyo*), the Switch will be slow as the transition from emptiness to balance occurs.

The Tsubo

The amount of pressure you apply depends on the state of the muscle, flesh and meridian energy. A person with well-toned muscles and a generally balanced energy system might feel good about receiving deeper pressure, whereas an unfit person would find this too painful. Ask your partner what they feel comfortable with. It also depends on the state of the meridians and pressure points.

The pressure points (in Japanese *tsubo*, meaning 'vase'), are areas of concentrated electrical charge along the meridians. Some tsubo will be tight and resisting (Excess), some soft and yielding (Deficiency), while others will feel vibrant and springy to the touch (*see* fig. 3.3). Think about each tsubo or pressure point as a vase. Place your thumb at the mouth of the vase and 'sink' into it using your body weight and *hara* (the belly, the physical centre of your body, thought of as the 'Ocean of Ki', referring to the storage of Ki in this area). Try this exercise to get used to working with your hara. Using a pillow, kneel on your hands (with your hands on the pillow), belly (hara) relaxed and your navel as your centre of gravity. Exhale as you gently transfer your weight onto your left hand and then onto your right. Experiment with applying pressure to the pillow by transferring your body weight. Do not use your arm muscle.

Practise this exercise before applying pressure on your tsubo as outlined above, being careful to avoid using muscle power, as this is sharp and activates the sympathetic system. Continue to apply pressure until you feel any tension dissolving and your thumb sinks further to the bottom of the tsubo.

Your pressure needs to be applied *perpendicular* to the body contour you are treating, so that you do not 'slide across' the tsubo by mistake. When you reach the bottom, there will be a deeper relaxation as the blocked Ki flows like water bursting from a once-blocked spring.

fig. 3.3 A tsubo in states
of Balance, Excess and
Deficiency

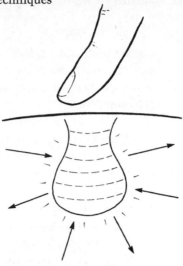

Balance: seven layers of energy of a vibrant
tsubo with Ki flowing

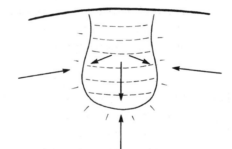

Excess: energy gathers to the tsubo causing a
stagnation of Ki – frustration of activity

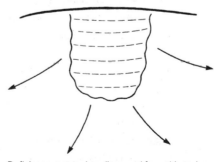

Deficiency: energy has dispersed from this tsubo
leaving a vacancy of Ki

Shiatsu for Women

Correct Posture
Correct posture is fundamental to giving good quality shiatsu. When you are comfortable and relaxed, your treatment will flow accordingly. We say, 'To create relaxation, you must come from a base of relaxation.' Some guidelines are:

- When kneeling, keep your knees wide apart.
- Keep your chest open, with the head slightly raised.
- Sink into your hara.
- Keep your elbows softly straightened.
- Bring your shoulders over your hands when applying pressure.
- Always move from your hara and minimize muscle tension.
- Regulate your breathing and apply pressure when your partner exhales.
- 'Lean' – never 'push' or 'force'.

Your Tools

Thumbs
These are your most important tools in giving shiatsu. Applying pressure to a tsubo requires that you use the flat of the thumb rather than the tip. Wherever possible, keep your arm held in soft extension (straight), to ensure that you use your body weight and not arm muscles, and try to have your shoulders come over the top of your thumbs as you lean into the tsubo.

Palms and Elbows
You may use your palm heel (the base of the palm just before the wrist) to apply pressure to a tsubo, meridian or muscle area. Just lean into this area as you would with your thumbs. Applying palm pressure covers a broader area and may be less sensitive for yourself or your partner. We commonly use the palms for treatment of the arms, legs and back areas.

Using the broadest tip of your elbow and/or forearm is sometimes very effective when seeking to apply deeper and more penetrating pressure to tense muscles of the shoulders, back and buttocks. Always work within your own or your partner's pain threshold.

Knees
Your knees can be a very useful tool, especially when treating someone larger than you. For example, by placing the knee (the contact point is just below your knee cap) on someone's buttocks and leaning into them, you can achieve a light or deep pressure over a broad area. With practice your knees will become as sensitive to feeling the Switch as your hands. Knee pressure is most commonly applied to the back of the legs, buttocks and sometimes different areas of the back.

Kenbiki – Kneading Techniques

These are basically skin-pulling, squeezing, pinching and rubbing techniques, which are very useful in activating better blood and Ki circulation to an area. These techniques go deeper than simply rubbing over the skin surface. The intention is to stimulate and release tension in the subcutaneous tissue (below the skin) and superficial fascia layers (connective tissue). Not only is circulation affected, activating the Heart Ki, but also your sensory nerves and the oil and sweat glands fundamental to supple and lively skin tone. The skin pores are activated and so react better to changes in the external environment.

These techniques are commonly applied to the back muscles, which tend to shorten and become restricted by tension. Since these muscles are predominantly 'postural' muscles – responsible for holding you upright and balancing your body – these restrictions cause postural imbalances, which in turn may affect your organ functions, especially those of the pelvis. Pinching and squeezing the muscles along the spine is both invigorating and relaxing and assists the trunk nerve communication to your organs (*see* figs 3.4–3.5).

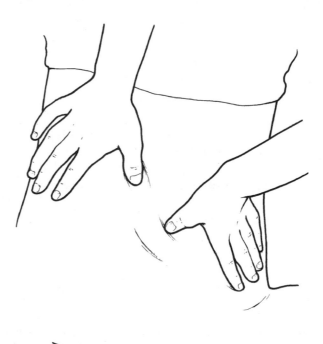

fig. 3.4 Kenbiki
techniques

fig. 3.5 Kenbiki
techniques

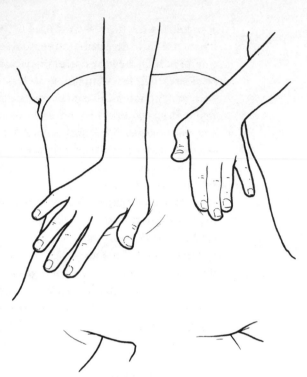

Stretches

Stretching meridians and, therefore, muscles and tendons, helps to rebalance fatigued and chronically shortened fibres and to stretch open blocked meridians. As a 'straightened' garden hose allows a better flow of water, so a 'knotted' meridian, with the surrounding muscle tissue in tension, will be relieved by stretching it. Stretches need to be held for at least 10–15 seconds, to allow the 'tissue memory' to change from chronic resistance to relaxation. Get your partner to lie on their back with their arms outstretched. Sit beside them and take hold of their palm and wrist in a gentle yet firm hold. Slowly and gently pull the arm until you feel muscle tension resistance. Do not go too far, it's just a mild stretch. Look at their shoulder and feel the shoulder joint open; 'thinking' into an area moves the Ki.

Stretching exercises should be repeated regularly to condition your body into a stabilized, relaxed condition (*see* the exercises on pages 121–8 in Chapter 7).w

Mobilizing the Joints – Rocking and Shaking Techniques
The Yin (Ki 'potential') is stored in the joints, which act as the connecting or communicating pathways and are also responsible for holding you

44

together as a complete unit. At the peripheral skeletal (arms and legs) joint sites, tsubo are more concentrated and the meridians come together in a confluence. Lack of movement causes the Yin to remain in the joints and so not be freely moved to the muscles. Stiffness in the joints and muscles indicates stagnant Ki in the muscles and stagnant Blood in the joints. Gentle shaking and rocking of the joints and limbs generally will allow a better flow of Blood and Ki through the area and encourage increased flexibility. Do the same exercise as you did with the stretching. but this time you can stretch and then add (at the same time) a light, shaking movement. Imagine that you are shaking out a beach towel, but shake the arm less vigorously. Amplify the movement in your mind with relatively little physical movement of the arm.

From a broader viewpoint, rocking has been a fundamental mechanism for relaxation from the time you were still in your mother's womb. Being rocked as an infant soothed you (sometimes), and even now, in times of stress, you may find yourself gently rocking your emotions into calmness. Gentle rhythmic rocking in your treatment will pacify the sympathetic nervous system, allowing deeper relaxation and the dissipation of toxic build-up in the body.

Try this technique with a partner. Lie on your back with your legs straight and feet close together. Have your partner take hold of your feet and *gently* 'rock' your feet towards your head, in a rhythmic motion of about one movement per second for 2 minutes. This acts to relax you and also to move the toxins by activating your lymphatic system (*see* fig. 3.6). You may feel a bit 'rough' for a day or so, as the toxins are released into your blood for elimination, but remember, it's better out than in.

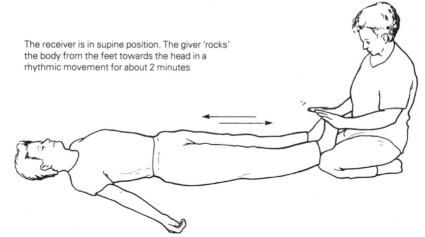

The receiver is in supine position. The giver 'rocks' the body from the feet towards the head in a rhythmic movement for about 2 minutes

fig. 3.6 Lymph drainage

Percussion Techniques

These techniques are used to create a vibrational resonance which penetrates the muscle tissue through to the bones underneath. The Kidney Ki controls the bone health, and the strength of your bones reflects your constitutional resource or Kidney Jing (the energy you were born with and further developed in infancy). Percussion techniques involve using either a loosely held fist or a cupped hand to actively tap various body areas (*see* the Do-In exercises in Chapter 7). This stimulates the Kidney Ki and the whole meridian system, as tapping also activates the meridians being worked.

Treating those 'I Can't Reach There' Areas

There are regular references in this book to the treatment of tsubo on the back and buttock areas. This is no problem if you have a friend to help out; if it is all up to you, then you might have difficulties. Help is at hand in the form of tennis balls or golf balls and an old sock. Take two tennis balls and insert them into a sock. Tie both ends of the sock, so that the balls sit together in the middle. Your 'tool' is now ready for action.

Lie down on your back with the balls placed on either side of your spine (where your Bladder meridian is located), and move them to the suggested tsubo site or anywhere you feel discomfort. There may be some initial tension, so breathe deeply and allow your body to relax and sink onto the balls. The balls will slowly mould themselves to your contours and stimulate your tsubo. Remain in this position for 3–5 minutes, or longer if it feels beneficial.

Single tennis balls can be placed in the hollow of each buttock to stimulate the reproductive organs more directly and relax the buttocks generally. Should you find that tennis balls are not penetrative enough and that you prefer a more 'positive' firm contact, use golf balls instead. Prepare them in the same way as the tennis balls.

Pain – What Is It?

People have shiatsu treatments for many reasons, most commonly for physical aches and pains. Emotional/psychological pain might not be as easy to detect, but this doesn't mean that it's not there and the 'scars' can be very deep indeed.

When you touch different points or areas of your body, you will encounter differing responses: some pleasant and others painful. Pain tells you that something is not right. Should you arrogantly or naïvely choose to ignore pain, you will no doubt suffer further and longer-lasting damage. In energetic terms, the pain is a symptom of stagnant Ki or Blood, or both.

When the pain is local, gets worse with the application of pressure and becomes sharp in response, then this shows an Excess condition. The pain of a Deficiency condition will be more widespread, subsiding with continued pressure and feeling like a painful but worthwhile 'relief'. In shiatsu we work with the pain. Application of pressure will help release the stagnation of Ki and Blood and gradually the pain will subside.

Tonification and Sedation

Using the body information determined from the pain response and speed of the Switch, you can then choose whether to sedate or tonify a meridian or body area. *Tonification* involves the attracting or gathering of energy back to an area deplete of Ki and Blood. It requires holding techniques where you wait patiently for the Switch to occur. This may also be achieved with gentle stretches, to relieve stiffness and improve mobility due to this form of 'emptiness' stagnation. *Sedation* techniques involve movement with brushing, percussion, stimulating and strong stretching techniques to disperse the stagnant Ki and Blood, allowing these to move to areas of Deficiency. So we:

- tonify Deficiency
- sedate Excess

Kyo and Jitsu Some tonification techniques might require the holding of a very Deficient (*Kyo*) area, at the same time as holding a very Excess (*Jitsu*) area, until the Jitsu softens and the Kyo becomes better toned.

Kyo and *Jitsu* are terms describing the movement of energy in relationship to the physical body. Deficient (of vitality) Ki is empty; Excess Ki is full, with too much vitality to be able to move – like a room containing too many people. They are thus relative states of emptiness and fullness. So:

- sedation – emptying/dispersing Jitsu areas
- tonification – filling/gathering into Kyo areas

The structure of the physical body acts as the 'border' or tangible, permeable container for forms of energy in motion and the energetic 'body' (*see* fig. 3.7). (Light and sound waves are less dense.) The physical body is obvious to our visual diagnosis, yet it contains other aspects of our interaction with our environment – our emotional, physiological and spiritual energies. These energies become more apparent through the way in which the physical body moves in everyday life. From this observation, we can see a psycho-energetic relationship developing. Changes occurring in the energy system will create a change in the more tangible systems of the body and its emotional and psychological condition. Physical symptoms, such as structural distortions, as well as psychological and emotional symptoms, are thus 'expressions' helpful in determining if a condition is Kyo or Jitsu and, consequently, the approach to effective treatment.

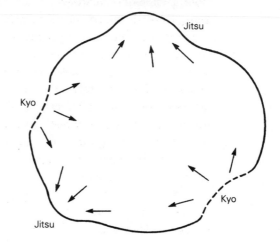

fig. 3.7 The Kyo/Jitsu
cycle of distortion

Some manifestations of Kyo and Jitsu:

Kyo	Jitsu
Empty	Full
Deficiency	Excess
Hollow	Dense
Soft	Hard
Deep	Surface
Wanting	Resisting
Hidden	Obvious
Cold	Hot
Lacks vitality	Excess vitality
Hypotense	Hypertense
Loose	Stiff
Collapse	Protection
Cause	Effect
Action	Reaction
Yin	Yang

Dispersed	Gathered
Non-movement	Movement
Chronic	Acute

These phenomena may be exhibited emotionally. For example, a person may be Deficient of Ki, lacking in vitality and perhaps very 'wanting' and 'hidden' in their communications. They may also be displayed in the physical appearance. A Kyo area may manifest some or all of the following: appear softer, puffy, collapsed; be lacking in resistance to touch; give rise to dull pain when pressure is applied. The Jitsu area may exhibit: a firm-to-hard texture; obvious resistance to touch; sharp pain with continued pressure.

Effects on the Autonomic Nervous System

When you are approaching a tsubo or meridian during a treatment, you need to consider the effects on the system as a whole, from both the energetic and physical viewpoints. A tsubo is an energetic confluence point reflecting the dynamics of the meridian and related *Zangfu* organs. 'Zang-fu' is a term referring to the differing functions and structural relationships of the 12 organs and meridians into two groups: Zang organs and Fu organs (discussed in detail in Chapter 5). The more 'solid' *Zang* organs produce and/or store Ki and Blood; the 'hollow' *Fu* organs activate the processing of the Ki and Blood and are responsible for the elimination of waste.

When a tsubo is in a state of Jitsu (Excess), this shows that there is a 'tension' prevailing, causing restriction of 'information' (Ki) flow. The same is applied to a state of Kyo (Deficiency). The relationship to the autonomic nervous system is as follows:

Jitsu causes	a *hyper* (overactive) sympathetic system
	a *hypo* (underactive) parasympathetic system
Kyo causes	a *hyper* parasympathetic system
	a *hypo* sympathetic system

In order to create 'balance' at a tsubo or meridian, we apply tonification or sedation techniques described earlier. The results of these, according to the nature of the imbalance, are as follows:

Sedation	pacifies the sympathetic system;
	activates the parasympathetic system
Tonification	pacifies the parasympathetic system;
	activates the sympathetic system

chapter 4

Two's Company! Shiatsu with a Friend

It is a wonderful gift to give and receive shiatsu. You are sharing a very close and personal experience, and this helps establish a greater understanding between people, whether it be between you and your lover, your child or a friend. It can help parents bond with their children, and friends and lovers resolve negative feelings, much better than words. Try it and see.

Before you start, it is important to think about your treatment environment. It should be clean, warm, comfortable and relaxing. So, no disco music or television blaring in the background. You may use gentle melodic music to calm the mind, and soft rather than bright lighting may also help. Some people like to burn candles and incense to add to the ambience (in Oriental philosophy, candles and incense help to 'cleanse' a space of negative influences). Do whatever feels right for you both.

Professional shiatsu is given with the receiver fully clothed, but when you are treating your lover, you can both choose to be dressed or undressed, perhaps depending on your location. Giving a quick shoulder treatment in a busy bus station whilst undressed may cause unnecessary complications!

Basic Frame Outline for Treating Yourself and your Partner
Prone Position

Preparation
- Before starting your treatment, always take a few moments to prepare yourself and your partner, who should be in Prone position (lying face down – *see* fig. 4.1). Sitting in Seiza position (on your knees), on your partner's left side, place your hand on their sacrum.
- Sit quietly, regulate your breathing, empty your mind, and focus on how your partner feels to you right now.

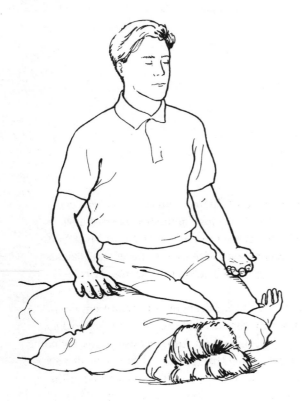 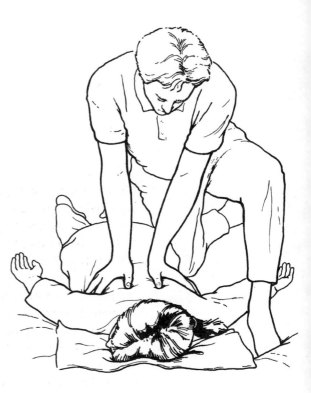

fig. 4.1 (left), fig. 4.2 (right)

Palming down Each Side of the Spine
- Measure two finger breadths/1.5 cun from the centre of the spine ('cun' refers to the measurement of a 'body inch' which is different on everyone and is the breadth across the pad of the receiver's thumb).
- Apply pressure with the heels of your hands close to the spine, with your fingers pointed to the outside (lateral) (*see* fig. 4.2). Start at the top of the Back (the posterior torso or back of your trunk), between the

52

shoulders, and work down the full length of the Back. Repeat three
times.

- Points to note: keep your elbows straight and use your body weight as
you work from your hara. Use the palm of your hands and apply pressure as your partner breathes out (*see* fig. 4.3).

Rocking the Back
- Kneel at 90 degrees to your partner. Place your palms in the valley (on
the opposite side of the spine) formed by the spinous processes (spinal
bumps) and the broad muscles running either side of the spine. Rock
the body with the heels of your hands.

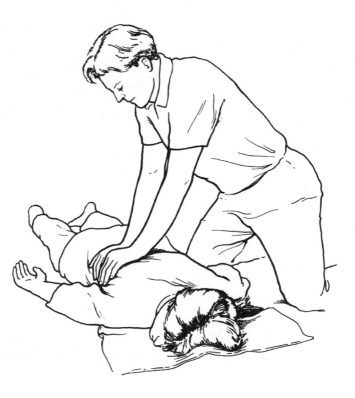

fig. 4.3

- As you rock, move your hands down the back, one following the other.
The rocking should be continuous and rhythmic.
- Repeat three times. Do both sides, first the right and then the left,
working from the opposite side of the body.

53

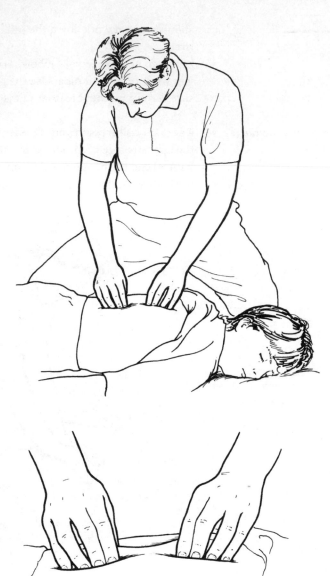

fig. 4.4

Rocking the Spine • This technique allows you to focus specifically upon the spinal column. The intention remains to rock, only this time the spinous processes are gripped between the fingers and thumbs.
• Applying a positive (firm) contact, the hands move along the length of the spine, moving it from side to side (*see* fig. 4.4). This loosens the muscles and stimulates the nervous system.

54

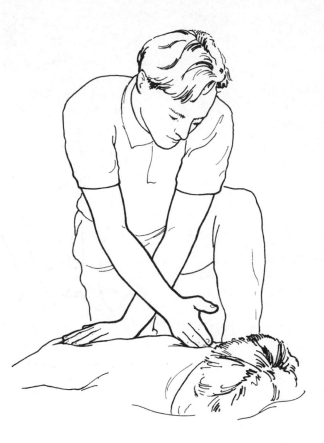

fig. 4.5

Sawing Action along the Spine
- Place your left hand on your partner's sacrum. Using the edge of your right hand like a knife, use this to perform a sawing action down either side of the spine (*see* fig. 4.5).
- Work both sides, repeating three times.

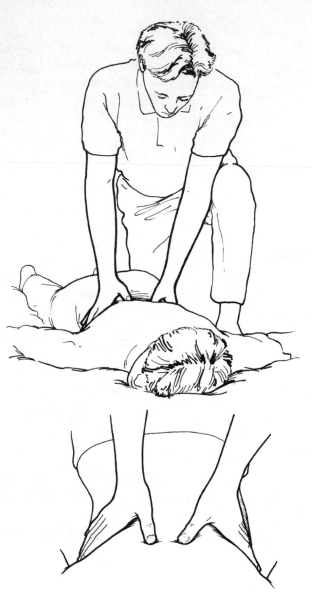

fig. 4.6

Thumbing along the
Bladder Meridian

• The inner Bladder channel (meridian) runs the length of the spine, two finger breadths either side of the midline of the spine. The thumbs are placed in the spaces formed between the spine's transverse processes (the horizontal 'wings' of each vertebrae). Run your hand along the spine and you will feel the undulations of the spinous processes (the vertical 'spines' of each vertebrae).

56

- Bring your thumbs sideways (laterally) two finger breadths (1.5 cun) from the depression between two spinous processes.
- Apply perpendicular pressure with your thumbs following the breathing of your partner. Start from the top of the back and work down to the sacrum (*see* fig. 4.6).

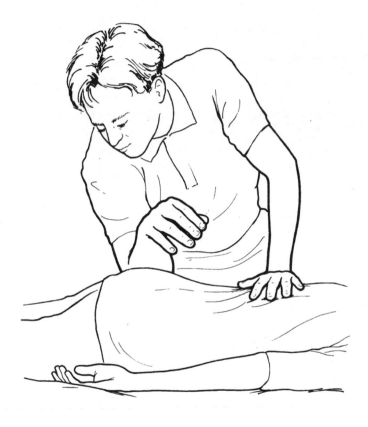

fig. 4.7

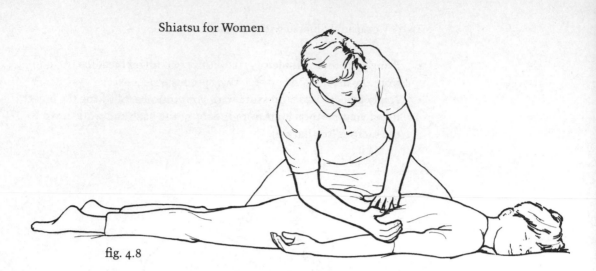

fig. 4.8

Forearm across the Buttocks

- Using the fleshy part of your forearm in a penetrating and rolling action, apply pressure across the buttocks. You may work both buttocks from the same side of your partner (*see* figs 4.7–4.8).
- Note the position of the listening hand and keep the hands relaxed.

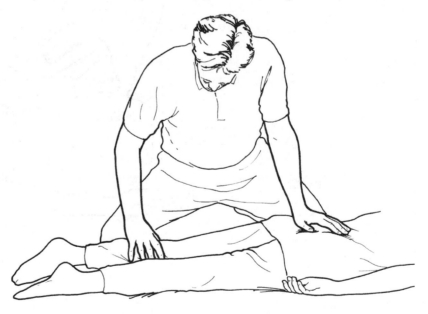

fig. 4.9

Palming down the Back of the Leg

- Adjust your position so that you can move down the leg without having to overstretch or become unbalanced. The listening hand remains on the sacrum or the buttocks area.
- Apply pressure with the heel of the hand or your thumb (*see* fig. 4.9).

58

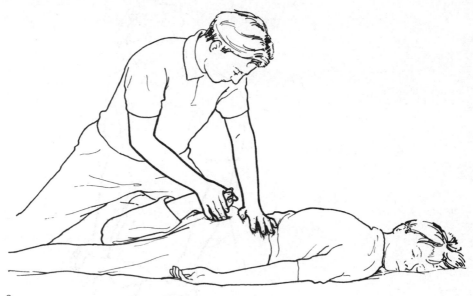

fig. 4.10

Stretching the Ankle to the Buttock

• Adjust your position to allow you to use your body weight to achieve the stretch. This also facilitates a smooth transition to the other side of your partner's body (*see* fig. 4.10).

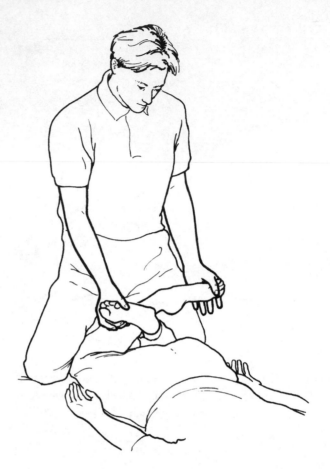

fig. 4.11

*Crossed Legs Stretch
with Ankles to
the Buttocks*

- Do this stretch twice. The first time, place the more flexible leg in front (nearest to the buttocks), and then reverse this position for the second stretch (*see* fig. 4.11).

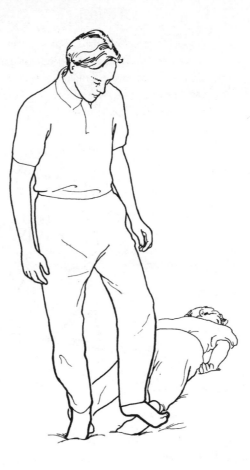

fig. 4.12

Walking on the Soles of the Feet
• Using your heels, walk on the soles of your partner's feet. Have their feet turned inwards and apply pressure to the soles, mainly with little or no weight on their toes (*see* fig. 4.12).

Supine Position
Assist your partner into Supine position (lying on their back – *see* fig. 4.13).
Once again, take a few moments of stillness to 'tune in' again while you
observe your partner. Place your right hand on their lower hara (lower
abdomen) and be aware of the tension or relaxation of the hara. Note the
breathing rate: fast and shallow indicates tension; slow and deep shows
relaxation.

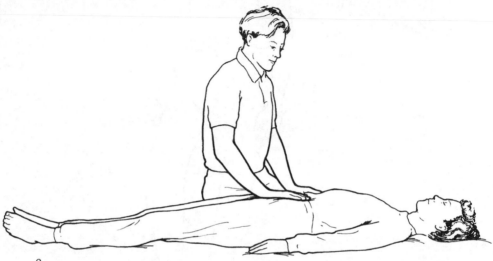

fig. 4.13

Tracing the Outline of the Hara
- Use both hands to feel and compare both sides of the hara. Start at the border of the rib cage, just below the breast bone.
- Move both hands out to the sides and then to the pelvic region. Now you know the main landmarks.

Anpuku Abdominal Massage
These two techniques are good for relieving menstrual pains and constipation (*see* fig. 4.14).

- Using two hands, one on top of the other, apply gentle yet firm pressure in a clockwise movement around the hara. You can then divide the hara into 12 segments of a clock face and apply finger-pad pressure at each area, making small spiralic movements. Where you find tension, go slowly from surface to deep as the tension dissolves.
- With one hand on top of the other, make a rocking and pushing type action, like rolling dough, from one side of the hara to the other, and pull back using the heel of the hand. Repeat until the hara relaxes.

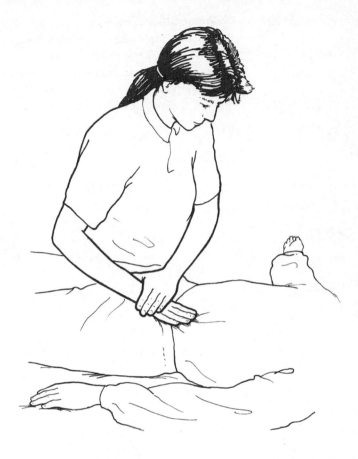

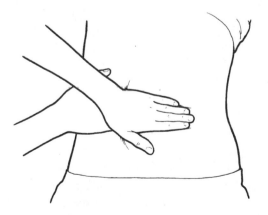

fig. 4.14

63

Palming down the Arm

- Your partner's arm is at 90 degrees to the body. Your listening hand supports the shoulder, whilst the messenger palms along the arm to the hand (*see* fig. 4.15).
- Avoid direct heavy pressure over the elbow joint.

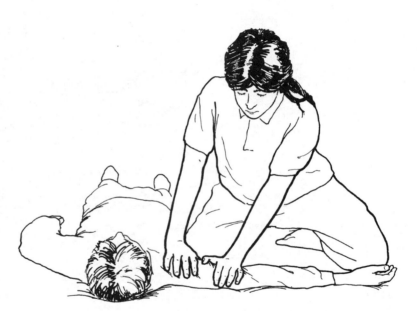

fig. 4.15

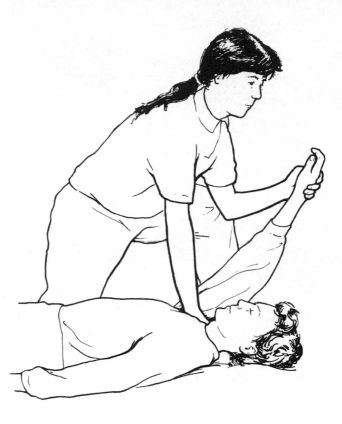

fig. 4.16

Rotating the Arm into an Overhead Stretch

- Hold your partner's arm by the wrist and support their shoulder with the other hand. Step forwards and rotate the arm into an overhead stretch. You need to apply pressure into the supporting hand at the shoulder before you step forwards, maintaining this pressure to ensure a strong stretch (*see* fig. 4.16).
- Step back, allowing the arm to return to the starting position. Repeat three times and shake and loosen the shoulder between each stretch.

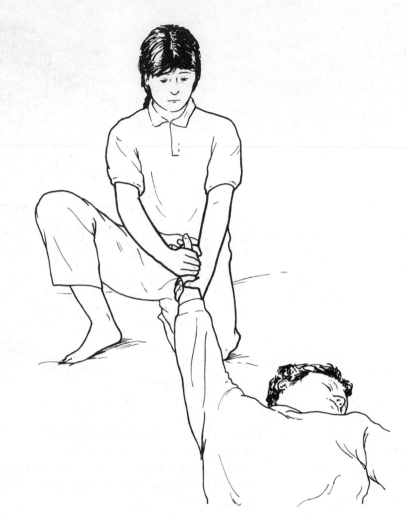

fig. 4.17

Overhead Stretch • Step forwards into the overhead stretch and bring your left knee (forwards knee) to the floor and pivot on it to face your partner's head. In this position, you can grip their hand and support at the wrist to achieve a maximum stretch by leaning backwards and using your body weight. Note the hand positions (*see* fig. 4.17).

• Reach down to take hold of your partner's other hand. Place both hands on top of your knees and stretch the arms by leaning backwards. Let go of the arm you have treated and make a transition over to the other side.

• Repeat the arm treatment on this side. Return to your partner's hara before proceeding to treat the legs.

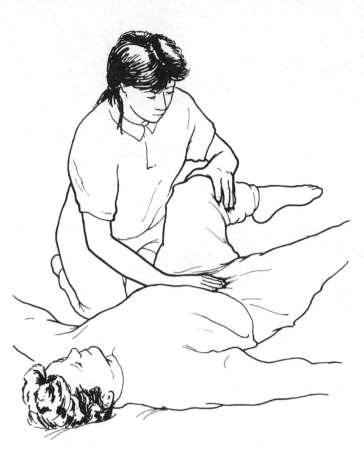

fig. 4.18

Rotating the Hip Joint • Your listening hand supports the hara, while the other holds the leg just below the knee. Use your body movement, not your arm muscles alone, to achieve the rotation, and move from your centre – the hara.

• Keep a fixed distance between your chest and your partner's knee, to ensure a balanced rotation of their hip (*see* fig. 4.18).

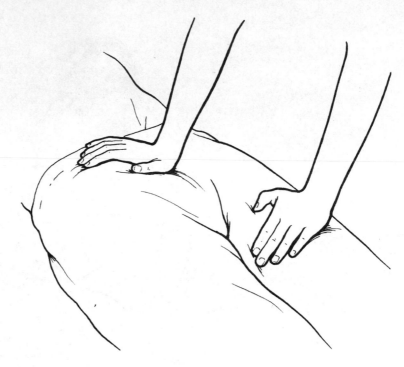

fig. 4.19

Palming down the
Outside Leg

- With your partner's legs lying straight, apply your palm pressure along the outside frontal edge of the leg. This is the Stomach meridian.
- You may need to place a pillow under your partner's knee for support and comfort. Repeat three times.

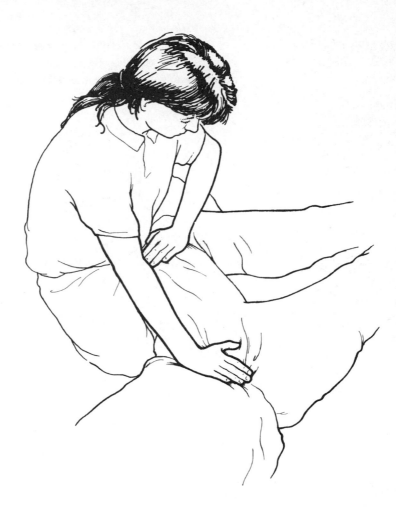

fig. 4.20

Palming up the Inside Leg
- Place your partner's foot to the opposite inside ankle, so that the leg is bent, exposing the inside leg. You will need to use a pillow or your own knee to support their leg to avoid groin strain.
- Using your palm, apply pressure from the ankle all the way to the groin crease. This treats the Spleen meridian leg branch. Repeat three times.

You may repeat this exercise in differing leg positions, which expose different meridians for treatment. Try bringing their foot arch to the opposite calf and treat in the same way. Then bring the foot arch to the opposite inside knee and treat in this position. Rotate the leg, stretch it out and move over to treat the other leg in the same way.

69

Sitting Position

*Kneading and Holding
the Shoulders*

- Get your partner to sit in a chair or on a pillow on the floor, as back support is necessary (*see* fig. 4.21). For this technique, you grip and hold the trapezius muscles (the muscles of the shoulders and neck) on either side of the neck.

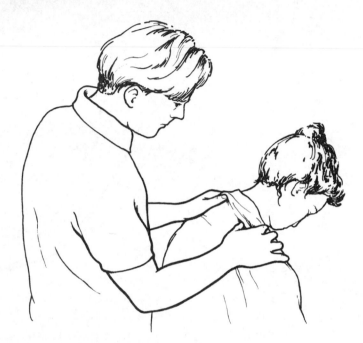

fig. 4.21

- Squeeze these muscles a few times, using the combination of your thumbs and fingers in a rhythmic 'kneading' action. There may be tension to begin with and this will slowly dissolve. Work within your partner's pain threshold.

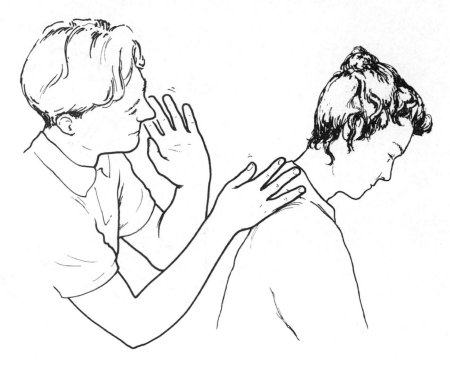

fig. 4.22

Hacking across the Shoulders

- Keep your own shoulders, wrists and hands relaxed and 'soft'. Use a gentle tapping motion (hacking) with the blade of your hands in a rhythmic motion across the shoulders and neck base.
- Increase the intensity and power of the hacking as the muscles relax and your partner's discomfort, if any, disappears.

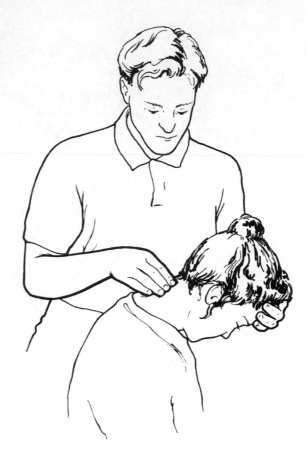

fig. 4.23

Squeezing the Neck • Half kneel at your partner's left side. Support their Back with your right leg, as shown. Ask them to relax and drop the head forwards into your left hand. Hold their forehead until you feel they have given up control of the neck.

• Using the fingers and thumb of your right hand, gently squeeze then hold the muscles of the neck, patiently working from top to bottom. Now repeat the same action with a faster rhythmic motion several times.

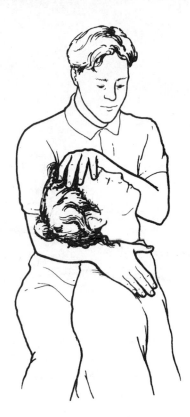

fig. 4.24

Stretching the Neck in Hyperextension (Bending Backwards)

- It is important to note that the base of the skull and neck must always be supported by your forearm, to prevent too strong a movement backwards, which could cause injury.
- Apply a gentle lifting movement with your forearm, as your left hand guides the head backwards onto your forearm. This has the effect of tractioning (stretching) the neck.

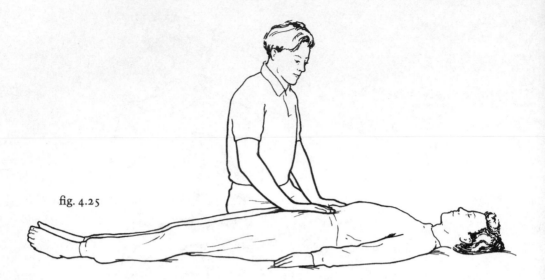

fig. 4.25

Completion • Get your partner to lie on their back again and rest. Place your hand on their hara and 'tune in' to listen and interpret the results of your treatment. The breathing and heart rate will have slowed down and the hara softened.
• Just 'be' with your partner for a few moments, then slowly dissolve your contact.

Additional Techniques

Kenbiki – Kenbiki techniques involve pulling, squeezing and pinching the flesh until
Improving Blood and the area reddens, showing the movement of Ki and Blood. Use a variety of
Ki Circulation these techniques over the buttocks, lumbar and spinal areas generally (*see* fig. 4.26 and pages 43–44 for method).

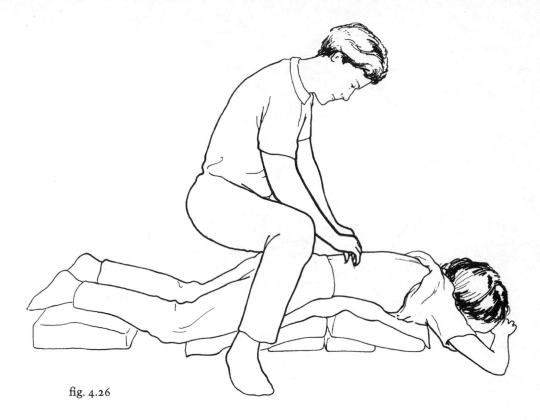

fig. 4.26

Opening up the Pelvis

- With your partner on their back, bring their feet together close to the groin, to open the pelvis. On an exhalation, apply gentle pressure on their knees with your palms, moving them towards the floor (*see* fig. 4.27 overleaf). Repeat three times.
- To strengthen the thighs and pelvis, apply some resistance to the knees whilst your partner (exhaling) tries to bring their knees together. Allow them to achieve this, but just create some effort for them. This is an isotonic exercise which draws Ki into the pelvis. Isotonic (equal tension) contraction involves the shortening of a muscle against a constant tension (force) with controlled movement.

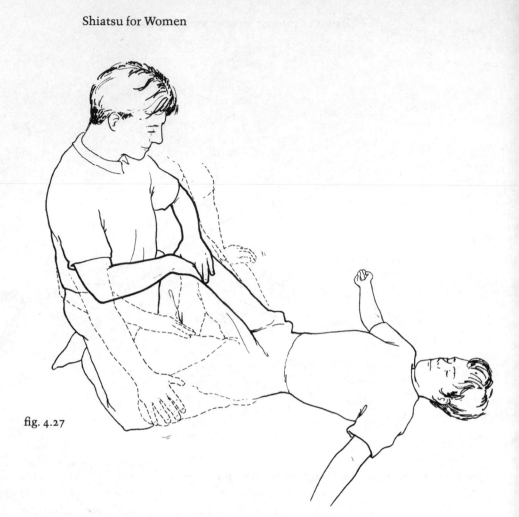

fig. 4.27

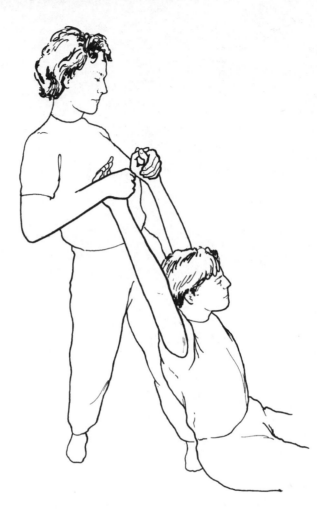

fig. 4.28

Stretching the Lungs • This allows for the greater intake of Air Ki. Get your partner to sit with their legs stretched out in front. Stand behind them with the side of one leg along their spine.
• Take hold of their hands, gripping around the thumbs and, as you both exhale, lift up from your knees and lean backwards until your partner feels the stretch. This stretch will open up the chest and shoulder girdle.

chapter 5

The Eastern View: Organs and their Energy Relationships

It would be easy for you to simply follow the treatment models set out in this book. You would of course achieve some success in this, but you will only progress further and create long-lasting changes if you begin to understand *why* you have your symptoms. Understanding organ functions and energetic relationships will therefore assist you in reaching this goal.

Zangfu Relationships

In Oriental Medicine we consider the importance of the whole body system as a cooperative and interactive form, functioning in harmony until such time as illness interferes with this balance. Even then, the body tries to organize itself to deal with illness in the most efficient and expedient manner. We must therefore consider the whole person in professional assessment or self-assessment. However, we are also influenced by more specific meridian and organ functions, which commonly are affected by or affect the reproductive system balance. For this reason, it is helpful to consider the 'personalities' of the *Zangfu* organs. The word 'Zangfu' refers to the 'Organs' in Oriental Medicine. In order to understand the variety of functions of these Organs, we shall discuss them separately as *Zang* and *Fu* Organs.

79

The *Zang* organs (Yin) are the more 'solid' and interior environment controlling organs of your body. We consider these to be vital to the balanced function of the system as a whole. The six Zang organs are the:

- Lung
- Spleen
- Heart
- Heart Governor
- Kidney
- Liver

Of these, the Spleen, Liver and Kidney have a primary role in your reproductive health. The Zang organs produce and/or store the Fundamental Substances – Blood, Ki, Fluids, Jing (the stored ancestral energy of your Kidneys) and the Shen (your Spirit).

The *Fu* organs (Yang) are the more 'hollow' and exterior environment controlling organs of your body and are the associated 'pairs' of the Zang organs. The six Fu organs are the:

- Large Intestine
- Stomach
- Small Intestine
- Triple Burner
- Bladder
- Gall Bladder

Their main function is that of elimination. They also have a secondary role in reproductive health, with the Bladder function (nervous system), the organs of elimination (Large and Small Intestines) and the Stomach (with its pathway through the nipples and ovaries) more directly involved.

Primary Organ Influences

Your 'wholeness' is a manifestation of the combined information stored in every cell. You cannot change a 'part' without affecting the 'whole'. In this concept of your bodymind, certain organ energetic functions have a more direct influence on your reproductive health. There are 'primary' organs considered more vital or essential to the maintained balance of your bodymind, and 'secondary' organs which assist the Burner in their work.

The *Primary* meridian/organ functions which affect the genitourinary system are the Liver, Kidney and Spleen functions. The Extraordinary

Vessels which directly relate to the gynaecological system are the Conception or Directing Vessel (*Ren Mai*), the Central Channel or Penetrating Vessel (*Chong Mai*), and the Governing Vessel (*Du Mai*) – *see* pages 93–6. The *Secondary* meridian/organ functions are the Heart Governor, Heart and Lung. The Three Burner function of the Triple Burner meridian is also intimately connected to the activity of the reproductive system (*see* fig. 5.1).

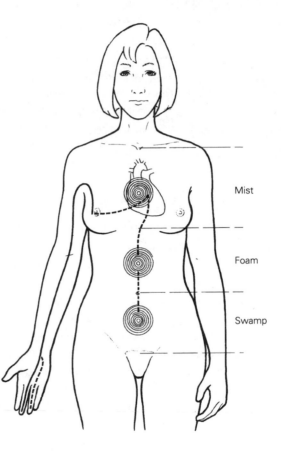

Mist

Foam

Swamp

fig. 5.1 The Three Burner locations

The *Three Burners* (the Lower Burner, Middle Burner and Upper Burner) are three body areas of the torso. Each area is regulated and controlled by one or a pair of Zang organs and supported by their 'sister' Fu organs. These areas also correlate to the cardiac, solar and hypogastric nerve plexi (nerve centres). If an organ is dysfunctioning, that particular body area and systemic function is affected and, conversely, if you are injured in one of these areas, the functions of the relevant organ are also injured.

The *Lower Burner* or 'Swamp' in Traditional Oriental Medicine, situated in your abdomen between the navel and the pubis, is governed by the Liver and Kidney functions. It also affects the 'patency' (smooth and unobstructed flow) for the Ki flow, and is much involved in the elimination of the 'impure' by-products of the energetic and physical systems. The *Middle Burner* or 'Foam', situated in the solar plexus area, is governed by the Spleen function and is involved in the 'rotting and ripening' of food. Hence the term 'foam', as in the juices of compost. The Middle Burner is therefore fundamental to the creation of Blood.

The Lung Ki or 'Mist' of the *Upper Burner* (situated in the chest area), involved in respiration, is also an issue because of its function of 'exchange and elimination' and the intake of Air Ki. This is vital to the Life Force of any organism, and to the quality of the Ki generally. The Kidneys 'grasp' the Lung Ki and integrate this into the body system, as this is a fundamental source of your vitality and is essential to the nervous system function.

Causes of Disease
There are three categories of disease in Oriental Medicine: External, Internal and Other.

The *External* causes of disease relate to the External Pernicious Influences of your environment and include Cold, Dryness, Wind, Summer Heat, Fire and Damp. These External causes tend to be closely related to changes in the weather and the seasons. They will not normally have an adverse influence on your health unless your Defensive energy (Wei Ki) is weakened and you are out of sync with your environment. It is through your breathing pathways of the mouth, nose and skin pores that these pathogens enter your system. These influences affect your organ function as follows:

- *Summer Heat* and *Fire* overheat the Heart
- *Damp* floods the tissue and overwhelms the Spleen
- *Dryness* hardens and dries the Lung and Kidney
- *Cold* chills the Water of the Kidney and tightens the Lung
- *Wind* penetrates the sinews and injures the Liver

The *Internal* causes of disease refer to disorders caused by emotional stress and its affect on the whole bodymind. Broadly speaking, there are seven emotions considered in Oriental Medicine. These emotions relate to differing organ functions (*see* opposite), as they may cause an excess build-up of Heat in their pertaining organ/s:

- *Joy* and *Sadness* make the Heart react erratically
- *Worry* and excess 'thinking' exhaust the Spleen
- *Depression* collapses the Lungs and brings lethargy
- *Fear* makes the Kidney Ki descend and internalizes the emotions
- *Anger* disturbs the Liver Ki, making it rise and flare with Fire
- *Shock* draws the Ki inwards and disrupts the Heart and Small Intestine

The *Other* causes of disease are: poor diet, lack of exercise, unhygienic living conditions, weak constitution, trauma, excess sexual activity or exercise, overwork, parasites, poisons, drug usage and being given the wrong medical treatment for your condition.

The Liver (Zang)
Function: Storage and Distribution
This is referred to as the 'Lion's Roar', an expression of the power and stamina of the Liver energy. The Liver is responsible for the 'spark' of Yang required to initiate muscle contraction and the reactive tension of movement. Muscle contraction and relaxation are fundamental to the successful flow of both Ki and Blood in the pelvic viscera (the organs of the pelvis).

The storage and distribution function affects the Lower Burner and the storage of Blood in the Blood Chamber (womb) of a woman. In Oriental Medicine, the idea is that menstruation should be pain-free and the flowing of the Heavenly Waters (blood) regular and without effort. Each month the Blood gathers in the womb and becomes Excess, the Blood Chamber then overflows and menstruation occurs. As a result of this there then follows a phase of Deficiency due to the Blood loss before the whole cycle recommences.

The prolonged functioning of the organs of reproduction is due to the stamina of the Liver Fire and its work as controller of the patency or smooth flow of the Ki throughout the body. Appropriately timed and controlled muscle contraction is responsible for your orgasm, menstruation and other eliminations. Symptoms such as lack of orgasm, weakened vaginal muscles, menstrual cramping and incontinence or 'dribbling' may be apparent with Liver Ki and Blood imbalances.

Sexual energy is a 'hot' energy and coldness in the hara can result in symptoms such as low sexual libido, poor internal muscle tonus, urinary incontinence, menstrual cramping or lack of orgasm.

The sensory organ for the Liver is the eyes. These reflect the 'life spark' in a person. Visual stimulation energizes the Liver and thus the sexual energy (fire), particularly when fuelled by the 'imagination' in both sexes, as Liver provides the fuel for 'ideas'. Imaginative and assertive in nature, the Liver's willingness to activate movement or lack thereof will help determine the Ki flow to the pelvis and the Three Burners needed for their reproductive energies. In the Orient they traditionally consider that the restful night phase restores the Yin reserves (Water), while the daylight activates the storage into Yang activity (Fire). During times of rest, the Ki returns to the Liver from the meridians for storage and body strengthening. It is thought, therefore, to be a sign of good health to awaken feeling sexually 'active' and that, for example, a man should awaken with an erection daily.

External Pathogenic Influences

The term 'pathogen' simply refers to any agent that can cause disease. The External pathogen of Wind may disrupt the Liver's patency ability and so create Heat in the Liver, causing the Liver Fire to rise and injure the Heart and Lung. Cold, particularly if affecting the Lung (which controls the Liver Fire) may indirectly congest the Liver.

Internal Pathogenic Influences

The Internal pathogens of repressed Anger and Fear (the Kidney Ki not nurturing the Liver in the Mother/Child cycle, *see* Chapter 6, page 106), and Depression injuring the Lung, creating lethargy, may injure the Liver and thus sexual libido, creating stagnation in the pelvis and Lower Burner. Because of the natural gathering and downwards movement of the Blood leading to menstruation, many traditional societies consider it harmful for a woman to have penetrative sex during her menses flow, as this forces the Blood upwards, creating stagnation conditions.

Treating the Liver
- Treat your Liver meridian generally by applying either thumb or palm pressure along the energy channel, or use the Do-In percussion techniques described in Chapter 7.
- Treating LIV 3 (*see* fig. 1.13, page 19) helps to tonify or sedate stagnant Liver Ki. If there is sharp pain or discomfort, it needs sedation with quick, rubbing movements; if there is a dull ache upon pressure, it needs tonifying by just holding the point patiently for about one minute.
- Self-treatment of your joints generally by the use of mobilization (movement) techniques will 'free' Liver Yin stagnation and allow better patency of the Ki. Refer to the exercises in Chapter 7 for help.

- While lying down, place your hands on your solar plexus area. Holding this respiratory diaphragm area relieves the Middle Burner to ease stress of the Gall Bladder, Liver and Spleen pertaining organs. Breathe into the area under your hands, taking long and deep breaths, expanding like a balloon on the inhalation and relaxing with the exhalation.
- When we rest, Blood returns to the Liver, before it is again mobilized with activity, which helps clear away Stagnant Ki and Blood. Aerobic exercise increases the Lung Ki which strengthens its Ko cycle control of the Liver (*see* pages 106–8 on the Ko cycle).

The Spleen (Zang)
Function: Ingestion and Digestion – 'Assimilation'

This is referred to as 'Nature's Lubricant', as it is responsible for the humidity and moistening aspects of the reproductive system and the quality of the interstitial fluid and lymph. The quality of the Spleen Essence, derived from Gu Ki (food and drink sources), affects the overall quality of the Blood. The Spleen energy creates the Dampness necessary for hydration of the body tissues. Both an Excess and a Deficiency of Damp will injure the system; the correct balance of heat and moisture achieves optimum Yin/Yang balance. The fluids for maintaining and nurturing the ovaries and the ovum in the graffian follicles (minute sacs in the structure of an ovary containing the ovum) are governed by good quality Spleen Ki.

The environment of the pelvic viscera in particular is dependent on balanced humidity control. The genital area needs to be warm and moist. Body humidity is more obviously expressed in the areas of the genitals and the armpits. The hair in these areas helps to maintain the moist, warm environment (so do not shave your armpits). Heat disorders injure the tissue and may create inflammations leading to scar tissue formation and Ki stagnation. For this reason, avoid tight fitting and synthetic underwear or clothing. Conversely, lack of support and the entering of Cold will damage the female genitalia. So wear comfortable cotton underwear to avoid the static electrical interference of synthetic materials.

Another function of the Spleen is to 'raise and support' your body Ki. It is responsible for maintaining the 'contours and curves' of the body: the muscle definition. Any sagging, collapse, swelling, or other loss of the body contours is, therefore, a reflection of Spleen Deficiency. The Spleen is also in charge of the transformation and 'regulation' of the Ki. So along with the 'curves' comes the control of the regularity of the body's 'rhythms', the most apparent of which is the menstrual cycle.

External Pathogenic
Influences

The External pathogen of Damp will injure the environmental control of the reproductive organs. The initial signs are related to the menstrual cycle, but continued untreated symptoms may lead to infertility. We consider that the Earth Element (*see* pages 104–5), especially the Spleen, controls the quality of the 'flesh' or body tissue. The inner lining of the uterus, the endometrium, thickens with menstruation, awaiting a fertilized ovum for implantation in its blood-enriched walls. Like the 'earth' of the external world, the endometrium reflects the environmental conditions required to initiate and sustain a healthy growing organism. Like a newly planted seed, the ovum will not find a suitable attachment if any or a combination of the following conditions of the 'earth' (endometrium) prevail:

- *Dampness* – a soggy, marshy, cold environment with an excess of body fluids. This can be caused by a cold and damp external environment or lack of exercise.
- *Freezing* – a hard, solid resistance. This is caused by Cold and Damp, from a possible Yang Deficient or Yin Excess condition. Other causes include a cold and damp external environment, frequent chills, lack of exercise and refrigerated food (especially ice cream and iced drinks).
- *Dryness* – a contraction of body tissue with deficient Body Fluid and insufficient Blood flow. This is considered to be a Yin Deficient condition, caused by dehydration, drying and heating foods (such as baked flour products and dried foods), and may also reflect a Yang Excess syndrome when Heat conditions such as cystitis prevail and dry the Yin.
- *Heat* – either a over-humid or over-dry condition resulting in Heat and Damp or Heat Flaring, or Empty Heat with Yin Deficiency. This is caused by excess animal foods, spicy foods, a hot external environment, repression of 'hotter' emotions such as anger, pelvic inflammations and infections.

Internal Pathogenic
Influences

Internal pathogens of Worry and Anxiety will stress the Spleen function. Worrying about your appearance and how the world sees you places great pressure upon the Spleen. Anorexia nervosa is an example of opposing views of subjectivity and objectivity of your self-image. The irregular eating patterns and lack of nurturing food and drink sources may damage the Yin. Thinking too much in work or study exhausts the Spleen Ki.

Treating the Spleen

- Treat the Spleen meridian generally by applying either thumb or palm pressure along the energy channel, or use the Do-In percussion techniques described in Chapter 7.
- Treat SP 6 and SP 9 (*see* fig. 1.5, page 13) to help tonify or sedate stagnant Spleen Ki (holding or stimulating accordingly).
- Hold the solar plexus area to relieve the Middle Burner and ease stress of the Spleen pertaining organ as you did for the Liver and Gall Bladder.
- Stimulate CV 1 (*see* fig.1.14, page 20) at the root of the pelvis to aid muscular support for the pelvic viscera.
- Place a tennis ball under each buttock as you lie on your back, and allow your weight to sink onto the balls. Locate a sensitive area and remain with this point for 2–3 minutes, until it relaxes.
- Stimulate the blood circulation in the buttocks and abdomen by using the Do-In percussion techniques described in Chapter 7.
- Get your partner to do the following Kenbiki techniques on your back, sacrum and buttocks areas:

Using the edges of both hands, rub vigorously along the sides of the spine.
Using the thumb and index finger, pinch the flesh on either side of the spine several times.
Pinch the flesh over the spine itself to stimulate the Governing Vessel channel.
Using the palm of the hand, rub vigorously over the sacrum and buttocks.

The Kidney (Zang)
Function: Purification and Regulation
This is referred to as the 'Master energy'. The Kidneys store the *Jing* (prenatal and post-natal Essence, derived from your parents and then your subsequent food intake and digestion or Gu Ki). The Jing is considered the source of all organic function and change in the body. It is the blueprint for your future growth and is the fluid-like substance which supports the body Yin. As a Fundamental Substance, the prenatal Jing is essential for your birth and future path in life, as it affects both your physical and spiritual being. It is a quantifiable source of vitality and is lost in the form of reproductive Essence, manifesting itself as ovum and sperm. Your ovum are a physical expression of the strong Yin of the body, which is exhausted gradually with ageing. Excess adrenal stimulation (through excess sex and fear-based

87

Shiatsu for Women

'adrenal' activities) and childbirth will also exhaust the Jing. These factors contribute to premature ageing, which is a sign of Deficient Kidney Jing.

The Kidney controls your vitality, Ki regulation, blood purification and 'appetite for life'. The Kidney is also the regulator of the Lower Burner and warms the organs and assists in the elimination of wastes via the 'waterways' of the eliminatory system. Thought of as the 'officials who do the energetic work', the kidney organs and the Kidney Ki provide you with the bright optimistic personality brimming with vitality and excitement about life. When the Kidney Ki is flowing well, personal relationships will be warm; you will feel and look energetic; stress will be controlled and you will not need the contribution of stimulants such as coffee, alcohol, smoking and excess sex to help your state of well-being. A stable sexual libido is a good indicator of the 'vitality' of the Kidney Ki.

Patterns of Kidney disharmony tend to be Deficiency states. The depletion of Jing and Nutritive Ki (Ki derived from food and drink), which help maintain and sustain the Kidney strength, is most common. We are not born with 'too much' Jing and, in our normal lives, we cannot take in 'too much' Nutritive Ki, even though we commonly eat and drink more than we actually need.

In relation to the reproductive system, the Kidney Yang ('activating' action of the Kidney) gives the 'spark' of fire for the reproductive process of the formation (ovarian stimulation) and propulsion of the ovum through the Fallopian tubes. The ovum is the more Yin, solid, slower personality, storing the framework for fertilization selection and foetal growth. The sperm is the more Yang, less solid, active partner, which provides the Yang 'spark of fire' to penetrate the ovum's protective surface. There are more Yin, slower sperm which take longer to travel to their goal but have a longer life than the more active fast-moving Yang sperm. These sperm will attempt to reach the ovum first, but have less stamina and a shorter life. The Yin sperm are more likely to fertilize the ovum if intercourse is immediately before ovulation; the Yang sperm will do so if intercourse is just after ovulation. It is thought that you can apply this as a method of predetermining foetal gender.

The Brain is also governed by the Kidney Ki and strongly influences the pituitary function of the hormonal system and, more directly, the adrenal function.

External Pathogenic Influences

The External pathogen of Dryness is injurious to the Kidney Ki. This creates a Deficient Yin (Water) condition, which may manifest itself as apparent Heat signs. In the long term, the body fluids, including the vaginal lubricants and 'water' quality of the environments for the ovum production, may become less hospitable to successful reproductive activity. The Kidney function also regulates the quality of the bones and its 'marrow'.

Internal Pathogenic Influences

The Internal pathogens of constant Fear and Anxiety stress the Kidney Ki. Fear is a hot emotion (Yang), often leading to an eruption of rising Fire, stimulating the Liver Fire to be expressed as anger.

Treating the Kidney

- Treat the Kidney meridian generally by applying either thumb or palm pressure along the energy channel, or use the Do-In percussion techniques described in Chapter 7.
- Treat KID 1 (*see* fig. 1.9, page 16), BL 23 and Ming Men (GV 4) (*see* fig. 5.2 overleaf) to help to tonify or sedate stagnant Kidney Ki (holding or stimulating accordingly).
- 'Projection' into the kidney organs 'warms' them and helps release any blockages. Rub your hands together vigorously until they become hot and then place them on your back at the level of the lowest ribs. Use your mind to 'wrap' the warmth from your hands around your kidneys and visualize light glowing from them. Try to feel them pulsing as the blood passes through them.
- Practise the 'lift and squeeze' exercises (on pages 146–7 under Strengthening your Ovarian Palace) to generate Ki and Blood circulation in your Ovarian Palace (the area between the umbilicus and the pubis).
- To activate the pituitary gland, hold GV 16 and In-Do (the point between the eyebrows) and 'project' Ki between them through the pituitary gland (situated behind your forehead at eye level) until you feel it pulsing.
- Use the Kenbiki skin-rubbing and squeezing techniques (*see* page 74) along the spine, to stimulate better blood and Ki circulation. This technique indirectly activates the Fire Element, especially the circulation function of the Heart, controlled by the Kidney in the Ko cycle.
- Stimulate the Reproductive Point in the buttocks (*see* fig. 5.2) using tennis balls. Place one ball under each buttock and lie on your back, allowing your weight to sink into the balls.

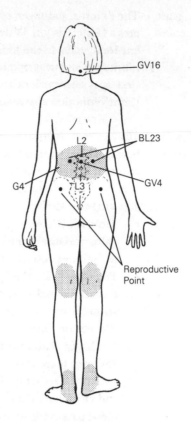

fig. 5.2 Location of GV 4,
GV 16, BL 23 and
Reproductive Point

The Lung (Zang)
Function: Exchange and Elimination – 'Transmission'
Through the intake of oxygen we embrace the Air Ki, the primary source
of life which is fundamental to harmonious exchange between the internal
and external environments of the body. This Ki-charged oxygen or 'Mist' is
infused into the bloodstream and reacts with the Spleen Nutritive Essence
to assist the Heart in creating the foundations of the Fundamental Substance of the Blood. If you are not breathing effectively, you are not 'living'
– this is your 'potential' being unused.

Acting as a protective layer both physically (skin) and energetically
as your Defensive Wei Ki, the Lung takes in Ki and 'exchanges information'
with the external environment. On the emotional level, your 'boundaries'
are supported by the Lung, with metaphors such as 'thick-skinned' showing this protective quality in the face of emotional abuse. Cold relations
with others are indicative of Lung Ki Deficiency, as clear communication
is restricted by fear of closeness. Insecurity, manifesting itself in the form

of 'gathering' material possessions and demanding the attentions of those around you, is another sign of Lung Ki Deficiency.

In Oriental Medicine the Lung is compared to 'the Prime Minister responsible for managing government affairs and keeping things in order'. Poorly oxygenated blood becomes polluted and sluggish, which sends Deficient Ki to the brain, causing a diminished response in the central nervous system, the controller of all the physiological functions. The Lung tissue incorporates the skin and membranes including the fascia, the connective tissue of your body.

External Pathogenic Influences

The External pathogens injuring the Lung Ki are Cold and Dryness. These damage the physical lung, which congests the Blood and Ki as it slows Ki movement. The Wei Ki is weakened, which has a knock-on effect on everything. When mucus hardens due to Ki stagnation, this leads to Blood stagnation, restricted respiration and Ki flow.

Internal Pathogenic Influences

As the Lung is regulated by the Upper Burner (the centre of Ki of the chest) and communication is part of its nature, Lung Deficiency leads to imbalances in the Chest Ki. These may disturb the Shen, with the effect of low 'quality of life' and consequent introversion and rejection of support. Depression affects the posture and the 'lung slump', with shoulders drooping forwards, creating blockages in the chest and the pelvis as well as an insufficient Air Ki intake. This may manifest itself as cystic growths, adhesions, water retention, coldness, sluggish eliminations with mucus appearing in the stools, feeling 'unattached' to relationships or a poor sexual libido.

Treating the Lung
- Treat the Lung meridian generally by applying either thumb or palm pressure along the energy channel, or use the Do-In percussion techniques described in Chapter 7.
- The power of the respiration and 'openness' of the Lung, in both physical and emotional terms, will be enhanced by the Lung Starfish posture. To perform this posture, place two to three pillows on the floor, lie with your upper back on the pillows and your arms spread out, palms upwards. You may need a smaller pillow or a few books to support your head, but the head should be allowed to hang slightly to open your throat. Spread your legs to match your arm position. Remain like this for 5–10 minutes, then place one hand on your chest and the other on the lower abdomen. Inhale deeply for 5–7 seconds, hold the breath for a count of three, and exhale for 5 seconds. Try to feel both your

chest and abdomen responding to the breathing rhythm. Continue this technique for 10–15 minutes and try to do it daily. It is particularly good for relieving chest congestion.

- Apply mild-to-deeper 'percussion' over the whole rib cage – front, sides and back. This will loosen any internal congestion and make the lungs more 'productive'.
- Hold the solar plexus area to relieve the Middle Burner, to ease stress of the respiratory diaphragm as you did for the Liver and Spleen.
- Treat LU 1, 10 and 11 as well as LI 4 (see fig. 5.3).

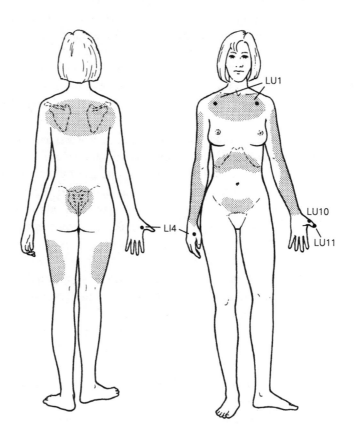

fig. 5.3 Location of LU 1, 10, 11 and LI 4

The Extraordinary Vessels

There are three *Extraordinary Vessels* of energy which create a circuit sometimes called the *Central Channel* (*Chong Mai*) or *Spiritual Channel* (*Mai* in Chinese refers to the vertical channels of the body). This Central Channel has two exterior aspects: the *Conception Vessel* or *Ren Mai* (Yin) and the *Governing Vessel* or *Du Mai* (Yang). These play an important role in regulating and governing the meridian system. As with most Oriental

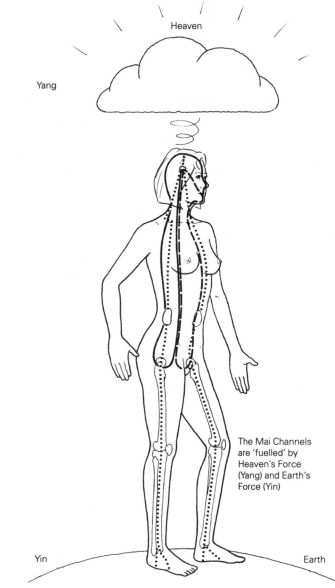

Heaven

Yang

The Mai Channels are 'fuelled' by Heaven's Force (Yang) and Earth's Force (Yin)

Yin

Earth

fig. 5.4
A woman standing between Heaven and Earth with Ki activating the five Mai Channels

93

theories of energy, these vessels are not separate from, nor are they the same as, the 12 classical meridians. They are the polar representations of Heaven and Earth in the physical and spiritual form (*see* fig. 5.4). (According to Oriental thinking, *Heaven* is an expression of the cosmos, more vibrational (not dense) in nature, and the source of Yang. *Earth* is the more dense expression of energy as it moves from intangible to tangible; it is the Yin nature and the 'soil' of life nurtured by the sun of Heaven.)

The 12 classical organ meridians receive energy from and give excess into these vessels, according to the body's requirements. It is at these central path crossing points in the body that the bilateral aspects of the organ meridians meet one another, forming a continuous energy flow. The Conception Vessel and Governing Vessel act as regulators of the overall body Ki and Blood.

These vessels enter the internal environment of the body at the mouth, meet at the mid-brain area (thalamus) and become a central 'staff' of power; they form the core of the energy system, strongly affecting your spiritual state (Yang) and the connection to Heaven. Placing the tongue on the roof of the mouth during meditation and breathing exercises stimulates the internal connection of the Central Channel, by completing the circuit of these two vessels connecting Heaven and Earth.

Central Channel (Chong Mai)

This is the internal pathway and the more Yin of these vessels. It governs and controls its son and daughter, the Du Mai and Ren Mai. As the controller of the Yin/Yang balance, the *Central Channel* acts like a computer internal hard disk or unconscious brain, storing both physical and metaphysical information. All events in this life (and perhaps past lives) are stored in this memory bank. Past traumas and happiness exists like a shadow, always in the background, awaiting revival when opportunity arises. Some 'memories' inhibit your potential and prevent your progressing with the fullness of life. Fear creates resistance to taking the risk of 'change'. By treating the Chong Mai, through the Du and Ren Mai, you can dissolve the inhibitions limiting your potential.

The Chong Mai internal pathway goes from your perineum (between the anus and the genitals), where it connects with the other two vessels, through your uterus to connect with your stomach on its way to the thalamus 'confluence' (the focal point where these streams of energy meet) with the Du and Ren Mai Vessels. In Oriental Medicine the uterus is referred to as a 'curious' organ, because it does not specifically form part of the meridian system. It is also called 'The Palace of the Child'. This internal connection between the uterus and the stomach may be a factor for the associated nausea of pregnancy and some stages of your menstrual cycle.

External Pathogenic Influences	Because this vessel regulates the Yin and Yang, it may be influenced by various External pathogens when these become chronic patterns leading to degenerative disorders such as AIDS.

Internal Pathogenic Influences	Because this vessel is the 'executive' controlling and regulating the whole energy system, it reflects and is influenced by all events in your life. Dominant Neurological Patterns (DNP) are stored by the Central Channel and initiate the way in which you respond to any given situation. Behavioural patterns ingrained by parental training, such as not expressing anger and developed insecurities (never starting or completing things because of the fear of failure, for example) may all affect your everyday life and relationships.

Conception or Directing Vessel (Ren Mai)
This is referred to as the 'Great Mother Flow' and is the 'sea' of all the Yin meridians. The word 'conception' is rather a loose translation and it is better translated as the *Directing Vessel*, as it is responsible for the directing of the Yin throughout the system. This vessel has the strongest Yin energy influence and oversees the body's Water (Yin). As the name *Conception Vessel* implies, it also influences your ability to conceive on a sexual level, as well as how you relate spiritually within your environment. The Yin meridians have deeper branches connected to the Central Channel, which lies internally posterior to the Conception Vessel.

External Pathogenic Influences	Because this 'vessel' regulates the Yin, it may be influenced by various External pathogens when these become chronic patterns affecting one or more of the Yin meridians/organs.

Internal Pathogenic Influences	Psychologically, symptoms of disharmony caused by emotional distress may include difficulty in sexual relationships, low self-esteem, a tendency to be overly self-protective, difficulty in communicating with others, or spiritual unrest. Physically, there may be diseases of the genitourinary system, hernia, coldness in the abdomen, bloating of the abdomen, infertility, menstrual disorders, premature menopause, stomach pains, gastrointestinal disorders, bladder infections or heart related problems.

Governing Vessel (Du Mai)

This is referred to as the 'Great Father Flow' and is the 'sea' of all the Yang meridians. This has the strongest Yang energy influence and oversees the body's Fire (Yang). The *Governing Vessel* acts as the central support for the spine containing the spinal cord and, as such, greatly influences your nervous system and mental condition. The Yang meridians are connected internally to the Central Channel (Chong Mai), which lies anterior to the Governing Vessel.

External Pathogenic Influences	Because this vessel regulates the Yang, it may be influenced by the various External pathogens when these become chronic patterns affecting one or more of the Yang meridians/organs.
Internal Pathogenic Influences	Psychologically, symptoms of disharmony caused by emotional distress may include a nervous emotional state, emotional hypersensitivity, rigidity in thinking, a belief that your own opinion is best, insomnia, anxiety about life or unfocused fears. Physically, there may be pains along the spinal column, headaches, back pains, diseases of the central nervous system, intestinal bleeding, haemorrhoids, anorexia, epilepsy, multiple sclerosis, paralytic diseases or myalgic encephalomyelitis (ME).

Treating the Extraordinary Vessels

* There are no specific tsubo on the Central Channel as it is an internal channel, but access may be achieved by stimulating the Governing Vessel: GV 20, GV 16, GV 4 and GV 2 (*see* fig. 1.15, page 21). Lightly tap these points yourself or get your partner to apply holding pressure for you. This will activate the Governing Vessel, the Central Channel and the Conception Vessel via the internal connections.
* Sit cross-legged with the heel of one foot touching your perineum (CV 1), and then bounce lightly onto your heel while breathing deeply.
* Get your partner to tap along the length of your spine and then they/you can tap your sacrum to stimulate the Governing Vessel.
* Place your right index finger just above your pubic bone, and the left index finger at the notch made by your clavicle joining with the sternum (the sterno-clavicular notch). Press lightly at these points, while breathing and visualizing a line linking the two points.
* Place your index finger on the cleft below your nose (GV 26) and gently press for 10 seconds.
* Using the knuckle of a thumb, lightly tap the area between your eyebrows. This is useful in treating frontal headaches and also stimulates the pituitary gland.

PART II

chapter 6

Assessing your Health with Shiatsu

Maintaining Good Health

I am the source of my own health and well-being.[1]

Good health is similar to happiness in that when we have it, we are
rarely aware of it, and it is not until we lose it that we realize how important and precious it is. The most important thing to learn about good
health is how to maintain it. Many people equate health with remaining
free from dis-eases. A reason for this might be that the word 'health' comes
from the word 'heal'. To heal oneself is often thought of as freeing oneself
from dis-ease. However, 'heal' also means 'full of life' and health is about
feeling whole, with a deep connection to yourself and your purpose in life.
This means self-love and self-respect.

The philosopher Lao Tsu said, 'Man attains health by returning to
nature.' According to the classical Oriental textbooks, to live in accordance with Nature and follow the law of Yin and Yang is the best way to
keep the body and mind in harmony and live a long and full life.

Following the course of nature is still the best route…
    Sow the seeds, reap the harvest.[2]

So how do you obtain good health? What do you need to do? Health is a gift you give to yourself; healing and health come from within. Health cannot be forced upon you from the outside. Listen to your body and acknowledge that you are an expert with regard to your own well-being. Unfortunately, some of us choose to learn the hard way, and it is not until our body is in severe discomfort and pain, screaming for love and attention, that we finally give in and listen to what it has to tell us. Tune in to your monthly fluctuations within and the hormonal changes throughout the menstrual cycle and menopause. The more aware you become, the more easily you can tune in to your strengths and go in the direction of your talents and happiness. Healing and health involve a change of consciousness. Start to develop an appreciation for the person you are and an awareness of your physical and emotional patterns, so that you can then respond appropriately.

> Our purpose is to bring Divine Love, Beauty and Bliss
> into the world in a way true to each of us.[3]

Prevention rather than Cure

As stated at the start of this chapter, the most important thing to learn about health is how to maintain it. The stressful society we live in does not exactly support a healthy lifestyle and you need to take responsibility yourself for obtaining and then maintaining your health.

Stress Reduction

Your body responds to stressful situations with an increased production of certain hormones such as adrenaline. This increase leads to internal environmental changes (for example, increased heart rate and blood pressure) and physical activity designed to improve overall performance. However, at a certain level, these disrupt your ability to cope and continued exposure to stress often leads to mental and physical symptoms such as anxiety and depression, palpitations and muscular pains.

> Here's a two-step formula
> for handling stress.
> Step 1: Don't sweat the small stuff.
> Step 2: Remember, it's all small stuff.
>
> *Anthony Robbins*[4]

There are basically two aspects to stress reduction. The first one is *life-style modification.* This means consciously changing whatever external situations you can that cause you stress. This could mean changing your job, seeking counselling for relationship problems or reassessing your goals in life. Often it is simply about taking more time off and just generally adopting a more open attitude, no matter what you are doing.

> Take rest;
> a field that has rested gives a beautiful crop.
>
> *Ovid*[5]

The other way to reduce stress in your life is to teach yourself consciously and deliberately to *relax.* This often means a conscious cultivation through repeated practice. Daily, programmed, deep relaxation represents the most important element of disease prevention. The following relaxation routine should be practised every day and last for at least 20 continuous minutes. Deep relaxation is not the same as sleep and, to gain full benefit from it, it is important not to fall asleep *during* the relaxation (you can of course nap or go to sleep for the evening *after* the 20 minutes relaxation).

• Lie down in a comfortable position. Begin from the head and work down to the feet, allowing all your muscles to relax, expand, become heavy and warm. Centre your consciousness in the lower abdomen.
• Breathe in and out from this spot and centre yourself. This will help you to calm your mind and result in complete physical relaxation.

When you have established the habit of complete and total relaxation, you can use the above technique as soon as you recognize the tension building in your body. (Alternatively, you can use deep relaxation tapes with spoken directions which are available from most health-food stores.) According to Oriental Medicine, tension both creates and is the result of impeded Ki and Blood flow and leads to both Heat and stagnation in our bodies. Therefore the quicker we can let go of and relax such tension, the less likely it is that pathologic Heat and stagnation will accumulate within us.

Exercise Principles
A certain amount of physical exercise is necessary if you want to maintain your health and prevent disease. When you rest or are physically inactive, your Blood returns to the Liver from the periphery. When you exercise or are physically active, the Ki mobilizes the Blood out of the Liver. This

helps to sweep away with it any stagnant Ki or Blood and gets things moving. Since stagnation of Ki and/or Blood are the main obstructing factors in most chronic, internal diseases, you can easily appreciate the healthful and preventive benefits of regular exercise.

Some form of aerobic exercise also benefits the Heart and Lungs. Aerobic exercise is equivalent to opening the release valve within you. It blows off the steam of accumulated Ki due to tension and stress, while deep relaxation is like turning down the heat under the pot. The key to both is regularity and perseverance.

> Never give in.
>> Never give in.
>>> Never give in.
>>>> *Sir Winston Churchill*[6]

There is a time, however, when you should avoid strong, vigorous movement or exercise – during your period. Strenuous exercise during menstruation can lead to Blood and Ki leaving their 'path' and such erratic Ki flow might result in imbalances such as uterine bleeding or menorrhagia. Sexual intercourse is another activity you should also avoid during your periods, as this is thought to reverse the flow of Ki and Blood from down and out to up and in, which tends to cause the formation of stagnant Blood.

Dis-ease

Dis-ease is not an enemy to be destroyed.
It is a friend to be listened to and then transformed into health.[7]

Allow dis-ease to be a learning experience for your own self-development. Become aware of your weaknesses, be thankful to them and see them as guidelines for behaviour, not as things to feel bad about. Often our weaknesses just point us in a better direction and teach us how to take care of ourselves in a more nurturing way.

Diagnosis and Self-Observation

Diagnosis is an art form based on the study of the human form, nature and experience. The foundations of diagnosis can be easily learned and its intuitive aspect is inherent in all of us. Developing your intuition and learning to trust it, together with experience through study and practice, provide the basis for accurate diagnosis. We do it every day in our relationships: deciding about a friend, 'You look tired' is diagnosis.

Diagnosing yourself can, however, be a risky business. Firstly, your subjective opinion may be blurred by the way you see yourself, which may not be the same as an objective opinion by a second party. Secondly, if reading this book is your first experience of shiatsu and Oriental Medicine, then you are no expert. So, if in doubt, see a shiatsu practitioner or other therapist.

In shiatsu we use five methods of diagnosis:

- Visual
- Question
- Touch
- The other senses, including smell and sounds
- Intuition

We put all of these together and refer to them as 'listening' to yourself or your partner, whoever is the subject of the diagnosis. Truly successful diagnosis requires that you listen without being judgemental and remain *objectively* subjective. When you 'tune into' your partner successfully, you can let go of your 'self' and become your partner for a moment, feeling their Life Force just as you would feel the vitality of a fast-flowing stream when dip your hand in it. If you 'listen' and immerse yourself in their energy field, recognizing their strengths and stress becomes easier and fulfilling.

Signs and Symptoms

In shiatsu there is a distinction between what is a 'sign' and what is a 'symptom'. Overall, signs and symptoms are an expression of the 'whole' person, in terms of energetic and physical balance/imbalance. *Signs* are what the therapist diagnoses through visual, touch and question diagnosis. These are objective considerations and may relate to such factors as the dark puffy bags lurking under your eyes or the fact that you always sit almost on top of a radiator for warmth (this indicates a Deficiency condition). *Symptoms* are based on the information provided by you, the patient. Combined, these signs and symptoms give an accurate diagnosis and prognosis of the course of dis-ease.

The Outside Reflects the Inside

The two other main factors taken into consideration in Oriental Medicine are that '*The exterior reflects the interior*' and '*The small part reflects the whole.*' Therefore a close inspection of the external components of hair, skin, bone quality, muscle tone, body smells, complexion, the tongue, the posture and emotional expression all reflect the internal condition. Since no single part of the human body can live in independent existence to the whole organism, it is fair to consider that each part contains and may reflect the blueprint information of the whole system. This has become obvious with the advances in the processing of information from DNA samples of body fluid or tissue.

In shiatsu, the primary areas to which we look in the quest for information are the face (*see* pages 108–12), hara, back, tongue and the meridians. Different areas of your hara and back reflect the condition of your internal organs. By touching and sensing the quality of the energy on the surface of the body, you can diagnose the state of health of the internal organs (*see* figs 6.1 and 6.2). Looking at the different areas of the tongue will in a similar way give an indication of the state of health of different organ functions (*see* fig. 6.3). Usually we will look at a combination of some or all of these areas.

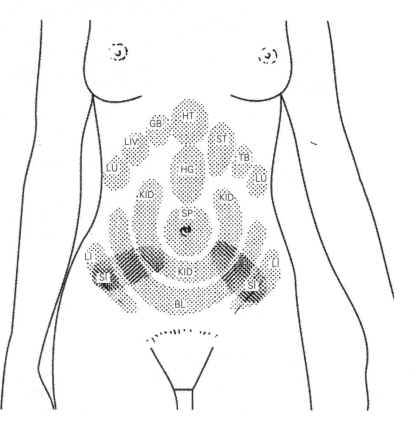

fig. 6.1 Hara
diagnosis map

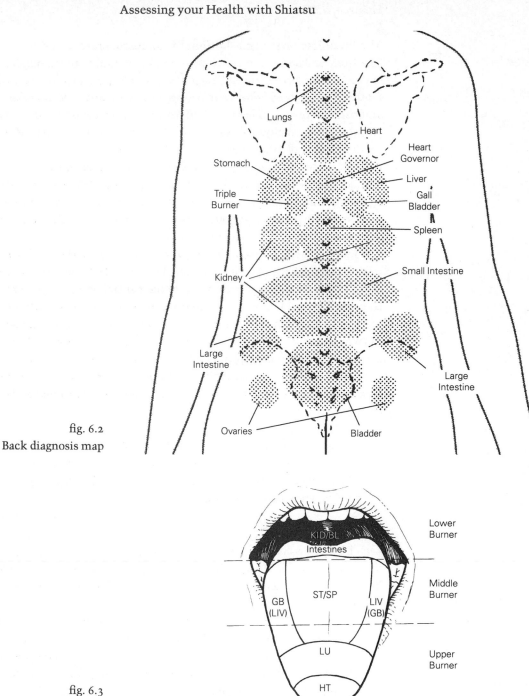

fig. 6.2
Back diagnosis map

fig. 6.3
Tongue diagnosis map

The Five Elements – An Additional Diagnostic Framework
The study and observation of Nature is fundamental to the understanding of Oriental Medicine. Yin and Yang describe the movement of energy, how it travels upwards and downwards or inwards and outwards. It is the core of the interaction of all natural phenomena and can be used to describe the physical and metaphysical essence of all things, from the structure of an organ to a state of mind or personality. Are you, or do you know the Yin-type person who is easy-going, likes one-to-one relationships best, is generally calm to the point of docility, is introverted and a 'thinker', particularly about 'spiritual' matters? Conversely, you may know the Yang-type person who is very physical, gregarious, extroverted, impatient, full of energy to do things and usually in a hurry.

Together with the theory of Yin/Yang, the theory of the *Five Elements* constitutes the basis of Chinese medical theory. The Elements compose the universe and, since you are a part of the natural universe, you are also composed of the Elements. You are the Elements, Nature is 'without' and 'within' us and each Element is a part of your being, just as it is a part of the world around us. Each Element has a character of its own and symbolizes different inherent qualities and states of natural phenomena. They constantly transform in accordance with the movement of natural phenomena and, in particular, with the interaction of your internal and external environments.

> The Five Elements are Water, Fire, Wood, Metal and Earth. Water moistens downwards, Fire flares upwards, Wood can be bent and straightened, Metal can be moulded and can harden, Earth permits sowing, growing and reaping.
>
> *Shong Shu*[8]

Each Element is connected with an emotion, a taste and a sound (*see* below) and is represented energetically in a pair of organs: one Yin, one Yang (these are the Zangfu organs as described in Chapter 5). In this way the necessary Yin/Yang balance may be maintained.

As Dianne Connelly says, 'The interaction of the Five Elements brings harmony and everything is in order. At the end of one year the sun has completed its course and everything starts anew with the first season, which is the beginning of Spring. This system is comparable to a ring which has neither beginning nor end.'[9]

Assessing your Health with Shiatsu

	Wood	Fire	Soil	Metal	Water
Negative Emotions	Anger	Excitability	Cynicism	Grief	Fear
	Impatience	Nervousness	Jealousy	Depression	Insecurity
Positive Emotions	Patience	Joy	Compassion	Positivity	Courage
	Humour	Calmness	Groundedness	Stability	Confidence
Tastes	Sour	Bitter	Sweet	Pungent	Salty
Sounds	Shouting	Laughing	Singing	Weeping	Groaning

Emotions, tastes and sounds associated with the Five Elements

Seasons of the Year

We all have our favourite and least favourite seasons. This distinction is usually a manifestation of your health condition and, in particular, the condition of individual organ functions. Someone who is more Yin will usually have less internal body heating, desire warm drinks, like to snuggle up in warm clothes and dislike the winter because the cold is uncomfortable for them. These are all signs of Deficient Fire (Yang) and will be linked to deficient Kidney Fire, the energy for warming you. You can achieve some insight into your own condition by observing your reactions to the seasons.

The Seasonal Day

Every day reflects the same seasonal changes that occur in the yearly cycle. Spring time is the period from pre-dawn to mid-morning; high summer is mid-morning to midday; late summer is the middle-afternoon; autumn is the late afternoon to early evening; winter is the full of night. Different organs 'peak' in vitality during the day. Should an organ become 'imbalanced' – that is, either in a state of Excess or Deficiency – then it will actually create some disturbance, either physically or mentally, during its normal 'peaking' time. For example, if you really dislike any disturbance first thing in the morning and find just about everything and everyone irritating, then your Liver is imbalanced. Good excuse, isn't it! We can relate the organs to the different seasons as follows:

- *Spring* – Liver and Gall Bladder
- *High summer* – Heart, Small Intestine, Heart Governor and Triple Burner
- *Late summer* – Stomach, Spleen and Pancreas
- *Autumn* – Lung and Large Intestine
- *Winter* – Bladder and Kidney

Ko and Shen Cycles

The different organ energies interact in a supporting and nourishing (generating) cycle called the 'Shen cycle', and in a controlling or restricting cycle called the 'Ko cycle'. As mentioned earlier, there are five constantly transforming Elements, each represented energetically in a pair of organs: one Ying, one Yang.

In the *Shen cycle*, each Zang organ – the Lung, Kidney, Liver, Heart, Heart Governor and Spleen – acts as the 'Mothering' and nurturing parent for the next Zang organ it enhances, which is referred to as the 'Child'. From this we may deduce that the Lung is the Mother of the Kidney, yet it is also the Child of the Spleen; each supporting the other in a continuous cycle (*see* fig. 6.4).

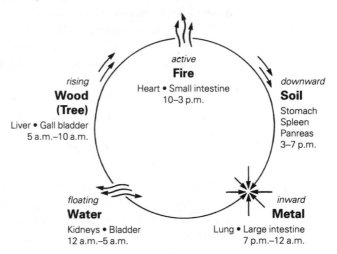

fig. 6.4 The Shen cycle expressing the Mother/Child relationship

The Elements are created and transformed dependent upon one another, as no part can act independently of the whole. With this is mind, we see the Shen cycle cooperation as follows:

- Wood acts as the fuel of Fire
- Fire generates the heat to create the ash of Earth
- Earth nurtures the growth and strength of Metal
- Metal 'contains' the movement of Water
- Water feeds and sustains the flexible Wood

In the *Ko cycle*, each Element controls another of the Elements and is in turn controlled by one. This is to ensure that a balance or equilibrium is maintained amongst the Five Elements. However, it may also mean that an Element may 'overreact' and 'insult' another Element. It is for this reason that the Ko cycle is sometimes called the 'destructive cycle', because the 'Parents' are squabbling for control of the 'Family' and confusion ensues. It becomes like an ego trip of your internal organs, each demanding the maximum attention and refusing to compromise. It usually ends with the whole energy system suffering and harmony being lost temporarily (*see* fig. 6.5).

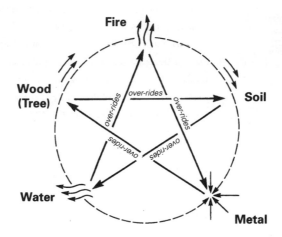

fig. 6.5 The Ko cycle

The interaction between the Five Elements in the Ko cycle is as follows:

- Wood roots and binds the Earth
- Earth covers and blocks the Water
- Water extinguishes the Fire
- Fire burns and melts the Metal
- Metal cuts and splinters the Wood

Understanding the Five Elements or Five Transformations of Energy is particularly useful as a diagnostic tool for determining energetic imbalances through observation and questioning. Many personality traits and habits can be seen to relate to different Elements and organ functions. Once an imbalance is understood, you are then able to design a specific treatment or give recommendations based on this information and understanding. For example, if there is an imbalance in the Water Element, you need to boost the Mother of Water – the Metal, especially the Lung Ki – in the Shen cycle and check that the Earth is not in Deficiency and drawing energy from the Water, or that the Fire is not flaring and overpowering the Water. If the Water is Deficient, boost it by treating the Metal (Mother); if it is in a state of Excess, treat the Wood to 'draw off' some of the excess and check the Earth and Fire Elements for Deficiencies (see figs 6.4 and 6.5).

Facial Diagnosis
The Microcosm Reflects the Macrocosm
The face is a microcosmic reflection of the macrocosm of the whole body and so reflects what is happening with your internal organs. Look at your face to determine your general state of health. A word of caution, however: do not become obsessed with your facial or bodily signs. Everyone expresses their condition in the outer appearance and this should be used as a method of realizing your strengths and weaknesses, in order to improve your overall condition. Here are some signs to look out for (see fig.6.7 overleaf):

- General facial puffiness is a sign of Spleen and lymph imbalance.
- Puffiness under the eyebrows shows Gall Bladder stagnation or congestion.
- Puffiness along the ridge above the eyebrow indicates sinus congestion and, therefore, Large Intestine congestion. The latter is a sign for general body congestion and indicates a Damp condition prevailing.
- Swelling at the side of nose is also a sign of sinus congestion and may indicate restriction of the bones of the nose (vomer and ethmoid) which affect the cranial bones (especially the sphenoid bone movements) and, therefore, indirectly inhibit pituitary gland function responsible for hormonal regulation. *To clear sinus congestion* try a sea salt nasal douche daily. Use lukewarm water in a bowl with a teaspoon of sea salt (dissolved); close one nostril with a finger and 'suck' the liquid into the open nostril and out through the mouth. Repeat this several times each side to soften the hardened mucus and activate discharging. In addition, you can also treat ST 3 and LI 20 (see fig. 6.6). Press upwards along the upper bone of the eye socket using your thumbs. Place your thumb against the roof of your mouth and push with a soft, upwards-directed 'pressing' motion against the roof of the mouth. This frees the nasal bones and stimulates the Conception Vessel of the mouth.

- Darkness at the inner canthus (the area between the inner corner of the eye and the bridge of the nose) indicates Spleen dysfunction.
- Horizontal lines across the top of the nose indicate Pancreas dysfunction.
- Temples showing oily textured skin, swelling, discoloration or pimples are all signs of Spleen Damp imbalance (*see* fig. 6.7 overleaf).

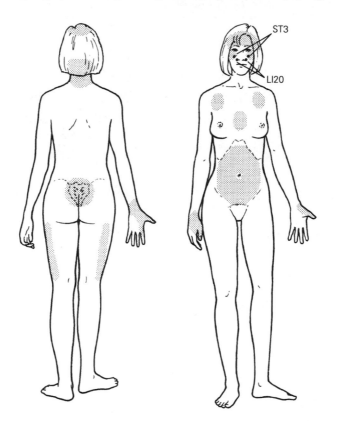

fig. 6.6 Sinus congestion:
point location chart

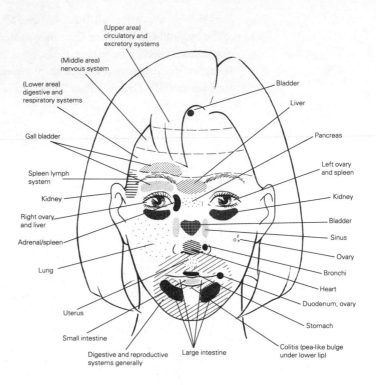

(Upper area)
circulatory and
excretory systems

(Middle area)
nervous system

(Lower area)
digestive and
respiratory systems

Bladder

Liver

Gall bladder

Pancreas

Spleen lymph
system

Left ovary
and spleen

Kidney

Kidney

Right ovary
and liver

Bladder

Sinus

Adrenal/spleen

Ovary

Lung

Bronchi

Heart

Uterus

Duodenum, ovary

Stomach

Small intestine

Colitis (pea-like bulge
under lower lip)

Digestive and reproductive
systems generally

Large intestine

fig. 6.7
Diagnostic face map

Facial Colour/Complexion
Facial colour expresses the health of your organs and conversely abnormal
discoloration shows disharmony:

- *Spleen* – yellow colour, sallow complexion, doughy and sagging flesh
- *Liver* – greenish yellow colour
- *Kidney* – blackish to blue colour
- *Lung* – pale or pasty to greyish colour
- *Heart* – reddish colour

The Eyes
The eyes are the 'windows of the soul' and generally reflect the Liver
'spark' of life:

- A pasty, dull eye expression reflects the energetic condition of the left
  and right ovaries respectively. Specifically, the left eye reflects the
  Spleen function, the right, the Liver. Puffiness or darkness below
  the eyes indicates Kidney Yang Deficiency.

- Pustules in the Kidney diagnosis area below the eyes indicate mucus congestion with potential for Kidney hardening (stones) – that is, Kidney Yin stagnation.
- Redness along the edge of the eyelid shows Kidney exhaustion.

The Cheeks

- A pasty or whitish colour shows sluggish respiration and circulation, which lead to a slowing of the pituitary function and the hormonal system generally.
- Persistent pimples on the cheeks indicate a potential for ovarian cysts on that side.
- Sporadically flushed red cheeks may indicate Yin Deficiency, especially when you have symptoms of night flushes or dramatically increased body heat during sleep.

The Mouth Region

The mouth area relates to reproductive and digestive functions generally:

- A greenish hue around the mouth is an indication of long-term stagnation and may be a pre-cancerous sign for the reproductive organs.
- A swollen lower lip shows Large Intestine sluggishness and poor digestion.
- What appears like windburn above the upper lip shows heat in the Stomach and may indicate a pyloric or duodenal ulcer.
- A horizontal line above the upper lip may appear after a hysterectomy or long-term dysmenorrhoea.
- Swelling or discoloration at the corners of the mouth indicates Blood stagnation of the ovary on that side.
- Hair growth on the upper lip on a woman is a sign of Excess, particularly Excess Yang, possibly even inherited from the parents, and indicates a strong animal food intake, particularly in childhood. This usually accompanies hair on the sacrum.
- Wrinkles around the mouth (like those that appear when you suck something sour) are a sign of potential infertility, where the womb is shrinking or has become cold and dry.
- A hardness on the point of the chin relates to reproductive congestion.
- Swelling all across or underneath the lower lip may indicate colitis.
- Cold sores (herpes simplex) are a general sign for dis-ease in the system and immune dysfunction (Spleen), often occurring at times of physical or mental stress.

The Chin
- A double chin indicates Spleen Deficiency and a lack of structural 'support', and may correspond with a pre-prolapse condition and hernias generally.
- Sagging jowls also express Spleen Deficiency.

The Hair
- Excess hair loss and premature greying show Kidney stress and dysfunction. Hair loss or discoloration towards the front may be caused by more sugar and chemically processed foods; towards the back, by more salty and animal foods. Premature greying is a sign of Kidney Yin Deficiency.
- Oily or dry hair shows poor Kidney Ki flow.

Body-Area Diagnosis
Different areas of your body reflect the condition of different internal organs. By diagnosing the state of a body area, you can gain information regarding the corresponding organ function (*see* fig. 6.8).

The Forearms
- Fatty nodules or cysts in the forearm may reflect fatty tissue or cysts in the breast on that side.

The Hands
- The fist relates to the heart; the strength of the *sustained* grip expresses the stamina of the Heart Ki.
- Clear undulations of the knuckles are a positive sign of the health of the heart; puffiness indicates hardening in the pericardium (the membranous sac protecting the heart organ).
- Clench your fists tightly until the fingers appear white – if the white is slow to disappear, it shows poor circulation (Blood stagnation). A purple discoloration at the tips of hands (fingers) is the Yin (Cold) trying to eliminate.
- If the hands are dry, this is a Yang sign; if they are wet, it is a Yin sign. Wet and cold hands show long-term Deficiency. Hot hands reveal a more acute Excess condition.

fig. 6.8 Body diagnosis
map

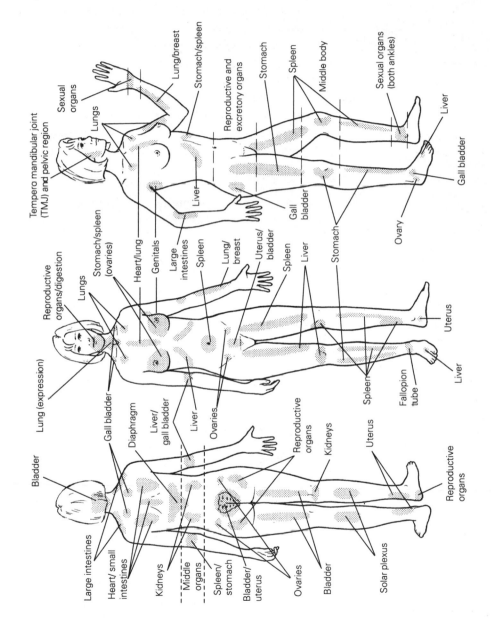

The Feet and Ankles
- Swelling, puffiness or discoloration indicates Blood stagnation generally and can be seen in different diagnostic areas. Discoloration becoming blue, brown and even yellow/green shows deepening stagnation in this order of seriousness. Check which meridian is discoloured.
- The inside ankle (medial) relates to the uterus; the outside (lateral) ankle relates to the ovaries.
- If the Achilles tendon is tight or swollen, this shows uterine congestion. Pain, swelling, discomfort or discoloration across the front of the ankle crease indicates distress of the Fallopian tubes.
- If the 'neck' of the big toe is painful, swollen or arthritic this indicates congestion of the cervix (the neck of the womb).

Treating any of these diagnostic areas by massage, or using your finger tips to apply pressure, will assist the relevant organs to improve.

The Pelvis
- Poor tonus of the muscles of the abdomen, buttocks and thighs shows poor Ki vitality and a weakened Spleen 'support' failing to define the contours and flesh. This is a sign of a sedentary lifestyle, commonly combined with poor diet.

The Skin
The skin can remain well elasticated and vibrant until you reach your 60s. The condition of your skin is a direct reflection of the functioning of your internal environment. When the skin and flesh is 'sagging' on the outside, there is 'sagging' on the inside. This may be related to specific diagnostic areas or it may be an overall condition.

- Healthy skin tonus will reveal itself as being smooth, supple, slightly moist rather than dry, and elasticated – that is, when you pinch and pull your skin, it springs back into place smartly. Another test is to vigorously rub or pinch an area of skin until it becomes red, and then see how long it takes to return to 'normal'. A Deficient condition will be slow to redden and slow-to-quick to fade back to normal. An Excess condition will be quick to redden and take longer to fade to normal.
- Loose skin which can easily be pulled away from the underlying muscle indicates Deficiency – lacking the vitality to 'bind' the flesh and indicating an existence of stagnant Blood and Ki with toxins not being successfully removed as waste. It also shows poor Spleen function and

weakened Wei Ki.

- If the skin is strongly bound to the underlying muscle and it is difficult to separate the two layers, this is an Excess condition. The skin will feel and look stretched tight.

Vaginal Discharge

Vaginal discharge is a normal process of lubrication, moistening and elimination. Vaginal mucus becomes more viscous and whitish in colour at ovulation. At other times, a healthy woman's discharge will be clear. Discharge might appear as follows and gives us information about our reproductive health:

- Clear mucus is a normal condition.
- White mucus indicates some mucus congestion and Cold and/or Dampness.
- Yellow mucus indicates a hardening of tissue and a Heat condition, probably combined with Dampness.
- Brown mucus indicates long standing stagnation and reveals Ki and Blood stagnation.
- Green mucus may indicate a pre-cancerous condition and you should seek professional advice.

Flesh Tone

- Pitting of the flesh indicates mucus collection and is found in areas where the flesh has swollen, as in oedema. Here 'mucus congestion' refers to Blood and Ki stagnation showing a Deficiency condition. It is related to Damp and indicates poor Ki circulation.
- Swelling around the ankles is an indication of Blood stagnation and Damp in the reproductive organs. If the swelling is more tight and the skin appears stretched, this is predominantly water congestion and related to the Kidney function. Determine the nature of the Damp by researching the other symptoms of Cold and Heat, as well as the 'eliminations' of urine and stool. Copious, pale urine and loose, watery stools indicate Cold. Frequent, scanty, yellow urine and dry stools or constipation indicate Heat.
- Puffiness on your sacrum indicates water or mucus congestion and Blood stagnation, with Cold and Damp in the Lower Burner.

chapter 7

Help Yourself to Health and Beauty

Feel Good, Look Good

When you feel positive about yourself and know that you are actively maintaining a healthy lifestyle, this reflects in your appearance. Knowing that you are doing the best for yourself and enjoying this process will bring a healthy glow to your skin, both physically and metaphorically. It's that old saying of 'Feel good, look good' – and it's true. You will soon become aware of the benefits of having greater vitality simply from the way people look at you: that 'spark of life' twinkling in your eyes will express self-confidence and security. This self-confidence will help in both your personal life and career, enabling you to release your potential and live life to the full.

Energize your Body and Tone your Meridians with Do-In Exercises

Your Ki is stored in the organs and other tissue of the body and commonly blockage occurs in the stored Ki of the joints. The joints store the Yin or 'potential' of your body; the muscles activate (or 'Yangize') this Yin to create action.

The term 'Do-In' simply refers to the 'Way of Exercise' and involves a combination of differing techniques to move your Ki. These techniques include percussion or tapping of the meridians and muscles, stretching exercises, and a wide range of breathing and movement exercises designed to improve your Ki flow. To create a vibrant state of health for yourself, you need to put in a little effort.

Awakening and toning your meridians ensures that you are using your full potential. By using the percussion techniques described, you can learn to activate the meridians in about 5 minutes of concentrated effort. It will take you a little longer the first time, but it gets much easier with practice.

Enjoying yourself is absolutely fundamental to successful and committed exercise. If exercise can become a stimulating and 'feel good' part of your day, you will have cleared the first hurdle.

fig. 7.1 Head, torso and leg percussion Do-In

Gradually create a regular routine of simple exercises that give you a vitality boost and help maintain a good state of health. Regular Ki-movement exercises such as the ones described below will activate the meridian and organ functions, allowing you to feel and look better.

The Do-In Daily Routine

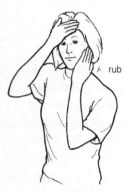 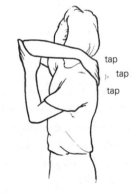 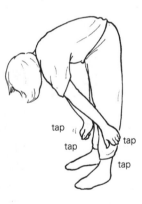

Head and Torso
- Stand upright with your feet about shoulder distance apart. Lift your shoulders and drop them a few times to take out any tension. Shake out your legs too.
- Make a loose fist with each hand and, keeping your wrists loose, practise a flapping-type movement with your hand.
- Gently tap the top of your head and then work your way all around the head, adjusting the percussion pressure as required. This wakes up your brain and stimulates blood circulation, which will also be good for your hair quality.
- Rub your face with your hands, as if you were washing it vigorously.

- Using your loosely clenched fists again, tap around the back of your neck, particularly where you feel tension. Using one hand, place the palm across the back of the neck and massage in a squeezing motion. Next massage and squeeze the shoulder muscles (trapezius muscles). The neck and shoulder area retain a lot of tension, particularly if you overeat at meals or overwork. Sitting at a desk all day also does not help, so take frequent breaks and *rub your shoulders.*

Arms and Hands
- Using your left hand to support the right elbow, tap across the top of your left shoulder (across your body) with the right hand (still in a loose fist), and up and across and down your back, as far as you can reach. Release the elbow, straighten the left arm in front of you, palm up, and tap from the shoulder to the open hand. Now turn your arm over and tap on the back of the arm, from hand to shoulder. Repeat three times.
- Working on your left hand, rotate and massage the joints of each finger by holding each between your right thumb and index finger. This is great to relieve hand stress and to help prevent arthritis and retain joint mobility.
- Using your right thumb, massage the centre of your left palm. This is HG 8 – the 'Palace of Anxiety' – which relieves general tension. Let your arms hang down by your sides and compare the two. The left feels light and vital and the right probably feels 'wooden' by comparison. So, would you prefer to feel light and vital or wooden all over? The choice is yours. Repeat the same techniques to your right arm and hand and then compare them again.

Chest, Hara and Back
- Tap across your chest – using either the loose fist or a flat hand for comfort – above and around the breasts and across your ribs. Massage your breasts (this is a good way of checking regularly for breast lumps), giving particular attention to massaging each nipple (ST 17 is located in the nipples), as this stimulates ovarian function and is also good for regulating or improving lactation in feeding mothers. Do this exercise daily to help maintain better ovarian health, which will assist hormonal regulation.
- Placing one hand on top of the other on your abdomen, make a circular motion around the abdomen in a clockwise direction, going down the left and up the right side. This follows the flow of circulation and digestion. Do this for about 1 minute.
- Place the backs of your hands on your back, just below the rib cage.

This is the area of your kidneys. Rub slowly to begin with, and then become more vigorous, until you feel warmth. This stimulates the Kidney Ki responsible for warming you and also aids an improved sexual libido as an expression of vitality.

- Bend forwards slightly and, using your clenched fists, tap from as high up the back as possible down to your buttocks, several times. Focus on the buttocks a little longer, until they feel relaxed. This stimulates the digestive, elimination and sexual organs by activating the parasympathetic nervous system.
- Using the back of your hand, tap over the sacrum bone and then as high up the bony structure of the spine as possible. Tapping the tail bone (coccyx) has the effect of decongesting the sinuses – so breathe deeply through the nose while you do this.

Legs and Feet
- Remain standing but with your legs wider apart. Keeping the knees slightly bent, start tapping (with the loose fist or an open hand) down the outside of both legs, from the hips to your ankles. Cover the whole of the outside leg. Now tap from the inside ankles to the groin, along the inside of your legs and thighs. Then tap down the backs of your legs, from the buttocks to the heels. Repeat this sequence three times.
- Sit on the floor. Focusing on one foot at a time, use a closed fist to 'knuckle' the sole of the foot by massaging the soles with the knuckles as lightly or deeply as you please. Massage the webs between each toe and then gently massage the toe joints, just as you did with the fingers. The toes are very important stabilizers for your balance and require loving attention to keep up such work. The leg meridian pathways mostly begin or end in the toes, so when you stimulate the toes, you are activating meridians at the same time. An example of this relationship is the symptom of gout which most commonly appears at the large toe, the start of the Liver meridian.
- Using your thumb/s, massage the area under each ankle bone, inside and outside. These are diagnosis and treatment areas for the ovaries and uterus: the outside reflects the ovary, the inside the uterus. Discoloration or puffiness shows irregularity in their respective functions.
- Take the foot in your hand and make a circular movement at the ankle to generally free up the joint mobility. Repeat this exercise on the other foot.
- To finish, gently and lovingly stroke your meridians by stroking all over your face, as if washing it, over your arms, hands, torso, legs and feet.

Self-Development Exercises: Meridian Stretches

These exercises are designed to enhance the functioning of your energy system by opening the meridian pathways to allow the free flow of the Life Force. Use the whole exercise routine daily or specific meridian stretches to alleviate imbalances in particular meridians. Remember, no one part of you can be affected without your Whole being influenced to some degree.

When you practise these exercises, it is important that you do not force yourself into the different stretching positions. Try instead to move slowly into each stretch, using your breathing as a guiding help, and give your body a chance to relax in between every stretch. Some of the exercises will feel easier than others – use this as part of a self-diagnosis, as it will bring awareness of where in your body you are holding tension and where the Ki is blocked. If you use your breathing in the way described and practise the exercises regularly, you will soon feel the improvement in flexibility and it will, of course, get easier every time you do them.

Exercise One:
Lung and Large
Intestine Stretch

- Stand with your feet slightly more than shoulder-width apart. Open up your feet so that your toes are pointed outwards naturally. Bring your hands together behind your back, with the palms facing backwards. Hook your thumbs together and spread your fingers out as much as you can (*see* fig. 7.2 overleaf).
- Inhale as you lengthen the spine by lifting your head towards the ceiling (as if it were supported by string). Exhale and bend forwards at the waist, keeping your knees softly locked. Stretch both arms back over your head, keeping your elbows straight. Stretch forwards as far as your body will go. Start to inhale and fill your body up with Ki. Breathe into your hara and imagine the Ki energy flowing from the centre of yourself out to your arms and legs. You will feel the stretch like a pulling sensation along the back of your legs, back and arms. You might also feel a line of tension or get a tingling feeling along the Lung and Large Intestine meridian.
- Exhale slowly and imagine Ki energy being released, allowing your body to relax. Repeat the breathing (inhaling as you fill your body up with Ki, getting in touch with the Lung and Large Intestine meridian, then exhaling and relaxing) another two or three times. Now slowly return to your starting position.

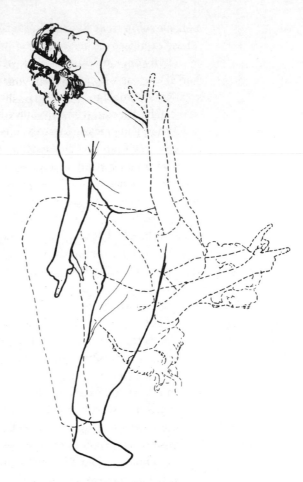

fig. 7.2 Lung and
Large Intestine stretch

Exercise Two:
Stomach and Spleen
Stretch

• Kneel on the floor in Seiza position (knees together, dorsal side of the feet flat on the floor), with your spine straight as in Exercise One. Place your hands behind you, with the fingers pointing forwards. Inhale and lean back onto your hands. Slowly exhale and gently push your hips forwards and up towards the ceiling. Allow your head to drop backwards (*see* fig. 7.3). Use the same breathing as in Exercise One: breathe in and fill your body up with Ki. You will feel a line of tension along the front of your thighs and all the way down to your second and first toe, as well as along your chest up to your throat. This line of tension corresponds to the Stomach and Spleen meridian. Allow yourself to relax as you expel the air through your lungs, then repeat the exercise another two or three times.

122

- You might feel that you can take this exercise a bit further. If so, try to come down with your elbows onto the floor, or even all the way down onto your back, with your arms stretched above your head. Be aware of any tension building up in your lower back as you perform these exercises. Remember never to push yourself – try instead to be aware of your own limitations in each stretch (*see* fig. 7.3).
- Come back up again to your starting position, using your hands to support yourself. Bend forwards and stretch out the opposite way. Use a nice loose fist and do some gentle tapping of your lower back, to ease up on any tension that might have built up in this area.

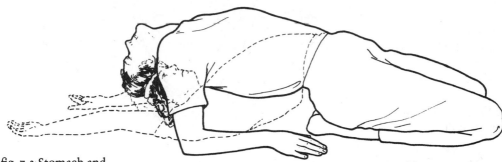

fig. 7.3 Stomach and
Spleen stretch

Exercise Three: Heart and Small Intestine Stretch

- Sit on the floor, bend your legs and bring your feet together in front of you (soles of your feet together). Draw your feet as close as possible towards your groin area by holding on to your toes. Straighten the spine as before. Inhale and lean forwards, keeping your back as straight as possible.
- Exhale as you bring your head towards the feet, keeping the thighs as low as possible and your elbows in front of your legs (*see* fig. 7.4 overleaf). Once again, remember not to force yourself in this stretch. Use the breathing to get in touch with the Heart and Small Intestine meridian. You are trying to bring your elbows, head and knees as close as possible to the floor.

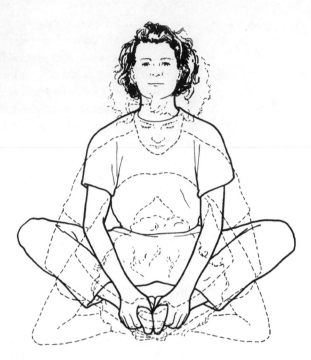

fig. 7.4 Heart and
Small Intestine stretch

Exercise Four:
Bladder and
Kidney Stretch

- To stretch the Kidney and Bladder meridians, sit on the floor with your legs stretched out in front. Straighten the spine. Pull your toes towards you, stretching the heel away. Raise your arms above your head, with the fingers clasped and the palms turned away. Look to the ceiling. Inhale, then exhale as you bend forwards stretching towards your toes. The knees remain softly locked (*see* fig. 7.5).

- Draw a deep breath and feel the tension from your waist down to your feet. Allow your head to relax down towards your legs and reach forwards with your arms and hands – feel the stretch along the back and in the arms. This is the line of the Bladder and Kidney meridians. Do not force the stretch as it may cause muscle cramp in the legs. Exhale slowly and relax completely before repeating the exercise a couple of times.

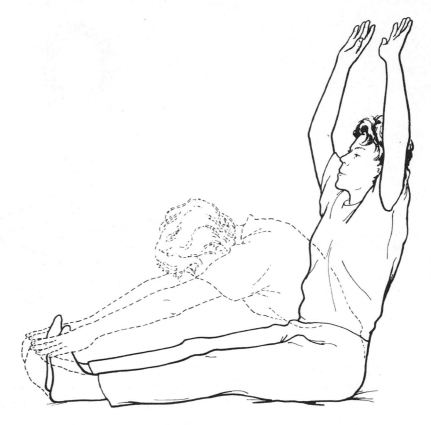

fig. 7.5 Bladder
and Kidney stretch

Exercise Five:
Heart Governor and
Triple Burner Stretch

- Sit on the floor with your back straight as before. Cross your legs, with the left leg in front. This is Tailor position. Without forcing, bring your knees as close to the floor as possible. Place your right hand on the left knee and, with your left arm in front, place your left hand on the right knee. Inhale and bend forwards while exhaling (*see* fig. 7.6 overleaf).
- Gently bend forwards and let your head hang down. Draw your body forwards and down towards your feet. Inhale deeply and fill up your body with Ki. You should feel the tension building up in your upper back and down the outside of your arms and legs. Relax as you breathe out and repeat the exercise two or three times.

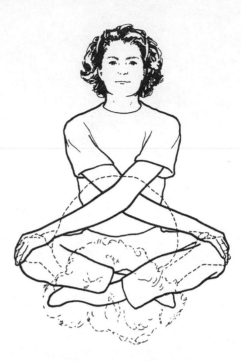

fig. 7.6
Heart Constrictor and
Triple Burner stretch

Exercise Six:
Gall Bladder and
Liver Stretch

- To stretch the Liver and Gall Bladder meridians, sit on the floor with your legs as wide apart as comfortable, keeping your legs stretched. Straighten your back as before. Clasp your fingers and stretch the hands (palms away) towards the ceiling (*see* fig. 7.7). Inhale and stretch towards your right foot while exhaling. Keep your toes pointed to the ceiling and face forwards as you do the stretch.
- Take a deep breath in and feel the lines of tension form along the side of your body. You should also feel the stretch along the outside of the leg you are leaning towards and down the inside of the opposite leg. Exhale completely and feel the tension go and the stretch increase. Repeat the whole sequence before returning back to the starting position. Inhale and repeat the stretch towards the left foot.

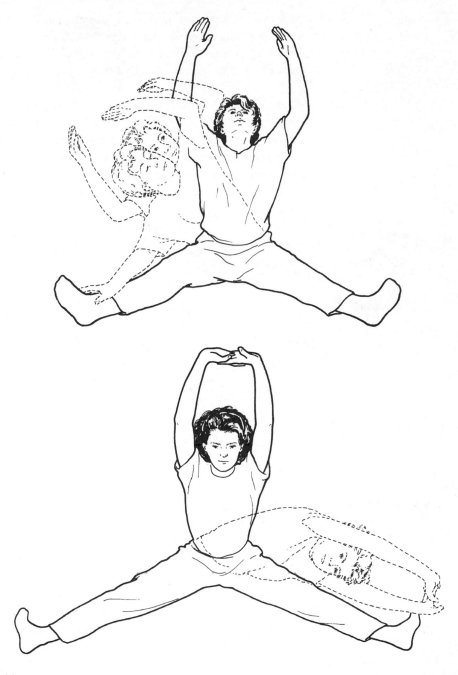

fig. 7.7 Gall Bladder
and Liver stretch

Shiatsu for Women

What is most important in all these exercises is to find the best position in which you can experience the energy flow along the different meridians. Practising the exercises regularly will improve your flexibility and you will gradually feel more at ease in the different positions.

Completion   When you have done all six exercises, lie down on your back and relax in the Corpse position (*see* fig. 7.8). Allow your breathing to calm down and your mind to relax and bring your attention to whatever is going on internally. Try to become aware of how the energy – the Ki – is moving internally. Hopefully you will experience a feeling of being alive and have a sense of energy circulating throughout, reaching and nurturing all different parts of your body.

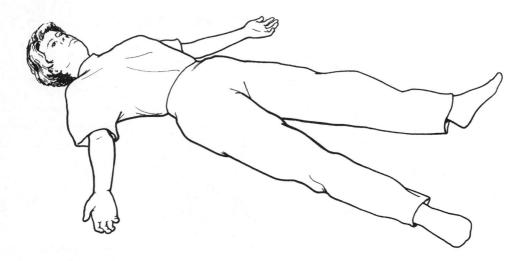

fig. 7.8 The Corpse
    position

I recommend that you combine these six exercises with the general Do-In exercises. Practise the Do-In routine, followed by the meridian exercises and a few minutes of relaxation and breathing to calm the system down. Try to make it a daily routine and you will soon feel the great benefit it has on your general well-being as well as your physical flexibility.

128

Stress – Who Needs It?

Breathing in Ki

When you breathe deeply and slowly, you take in a key source of energy – Air Ki. Your lungs are responsible for oxygenating the blood which gives you a 'Ki charge', as this refreshed blood travels to vital organs, moistening and revitalizing them. The largest consumer of blood in the body is your brain, the head of the central nervous system, which in turn sends messages to stimulate the organ functions. Deep breathing activates the parasympathetic (calming) nervous system branch, which slows the heart beat and calms the system. Conversely, if the Air Ki intake is low due to shallow, rapid breathing, the blood flow to the brain will be sluggish and the nervous system functions restricted. As a result of this the sympathetic (activating) nervous system branch will dominate. This will speed the heart and prepare the body for action, as in the 'fight or flight' response – stress!

It is your brain activating the nervous system in the first place that initiates the breathing cycle. A vicious circle is created, therefore, when poor breathing habits prevail. You need to make a conscious effort to breathe more deeply to break this pattern. Think about it – a more stimulated brain supports a more responsive nervous system and, therefore, a balanced body homeostasis (internal environment balance). Consider each breath as new life and vitality dissolving stress and anxiety.

'Mindfulness' Meditation Try this exercise first thing in the morning and last thing at night, to combat stress and help you enjoy a deeper and more recuperative sleep.

- Sit in a straight-backed chair with both feet flat on the floor or, alternatively, lie down in your bed, if this feels more relaxing. Some people prefer to sit on the floor with a pillow under the backside, to help keep the spine easily supported. Straighten your spine and tuck the chin towards your chest, but do not create strain. This opens up the spine and spinal cord, which will assist relaxation. Place your hands in your lap, the left hand resting on the right.
- Close your mouth and eyes and focus on the movement of the breath though the nostrils. Bring your attention to your abdomen, especially the area between the navel and the pubis. As you inhale, allow your hara (belly) to expand like a balloon filling with air. On the exhalation, suck in your abdomen to help expel the breath. Practise this for several breaths, as you may find it difficult to coordinate at first. Continue to breathe through the nose only. When you are ready, make each

inhalation last for 5–7 seconds, hold the breath for 3 seconds, and then exhale for about 5 seconds. Repeat this until you feel your body relaxing and becoming heavier as the tension releases.

If you find it difficult to maintain your concentration, try a simple meditation exercise as follows:

- Use one of the postures above. Keep concentrating on the movement of air through your nostrils.
- Visualize a blank cinema screen in your mind's eye, to avoid any distraction and give yourself a focal point. After each exhalation, project a number onto your screen, counting from one to ten in turn.
- Each time your concentration lapses and you find other thoughts prevailing, acknowledge that thought, and then return to the number one and try again to make it to ten without distraction.

You will probably find this a difficult exercise at first, but practice will make it easier and allow you greater concentration in other aspects of your life. The brain, like muscles, grows stronger with exercise.

The Art in your Brain[1]

Making a comparison between the Eastern and Western perspectives on health and healing can sometimes be a frustrating venture. Western medical diagnosis and treatment is based in science, with its rigid parameters and dualistic viewpoint. It is simply placed in terms of black and white, right and wrong – you have a disease which needs to be eradicated. This can be a disempowering experience for the strongest of people, as it means that when you have an illness, there is no self-responsibility, because it apparently comes externally and is therefore out of your control. Fear-based assessments also take away your own ability to listen to what your inner voice is telling you – that is, you can heal yourself, with help.

The scientific approach is centred in the left brain analytical functions and, therefore, promotes a logical and intellectual approach to designing remedial medicine. In Eastern healing medicines, the emphasis is placed on the right brain interpretation of illness and emphasizes the natural powers of self-healing.

Intuition and feelings of what is 'right' come from your right brain function. There may not necessarily be a logical reason why you chose to do something other than that it simply 'feels right'. In Oriental Medicine the practitioner has a wealth of anecdotal study and experience. This provides a strong foundation for determining the possible causes of dis-ease, to back up the greater power of intuition in giving successful treatment. If you ignore the intuitive aspects and simply rely on intellectual information, this will lead to a less effective treatment. So instead of identifying a person's weakness and designing your treatment on this basis, we emphasize that you discover the powerful resources still available and strengthen these. Release the potential and empower the 'person within'.

The Brain
Shiatsu is an experiential art form relying on your creativity and developing this will allow you to give yourself and your partner powerful and healing treatments. Anyone can study and mimic technique, but it is the initiation of your intuition that will release you to transcend the limitations of physical-based treatment to a higher level. Allowing your own creativity to blossom will give you the freedom to think of every new treatment as the best and most interesting yet.

The brain has two hemispheres – left and right – each controlling differing and complementary functions in your body and mind. This is a Yin/Yang balance. Physically, the left hemisphere controls the right side of the body, and the right hemisphere, the left side. The interaction between the two sides is continually adapting to deal with the needs of everyday activity.

In her book *Drawing on the Right Side of the Brain*,[2] Betty Edwards describes the 'modes' of the left and right brain function as follows:

> The Left mode is the 'right handed', left hemisphere mode. The Left is foursquare, upright, sensible, direct, true, hard-edged, unfanciful and forceful.
> The Right mode is the 'left handed', right hemisphere mode. The Right is curvy, flexible, more playful in its unexpected twists and turns, more complex, diagonal and fanciful.

The functions of the brain and its respective hemispheres create a crossover for the interpretation of information on differing levels. The *left* mode interprets more the 'modern' era of development of the ego, intellect, gatherer and aggressive protector nature. There is a developed or acquired intuition which is activated by life experience and is limited to the current life experiences and education with a cultural, religious and social basis. The *right* mode holds the evolutionary imprint inherent in all animals, most easily seen in the 'built-in' ability of a bird to fly. We too have this deeper or primal intuition, which can be resourced at will with experience.

The Power of Thought

You create your own reality. What you choose to think about yourself and your life becomes true to you, and you have unlimited choices about what you can think.

A simple thought has a significant impact on your mind, body and emotions. Positive thoughts such as joy and happiness, achievement and fulfilment, will produce positive results in your Being. Similarly, negative thoughts about resentment, fear or unworthiness, for example, will have negative results for you.

All your thoughts have responses in the body and also influence your emotions. Try this exercise:

- Close your eyes and imagine a place you really like. Maybe your favourite place in nature? A nice, sunny beach somewhere? Or your favourite corner at home? Your garden? Tune in to the flowers and smell the air. How does it make you feel? Relaxed? Happy? Think about someone you love and care for. How do you feel?
- Now bring yourself back to a situation when you felt really angry and frustrated. How do you react? Perhaps you were caught in a traffic jam and making you late for your appointment. What kind of body reactions do you get? Now, do you agree with the statement made earlier, that thoughts have power over your mind, body and emotions?

Affirmations

Affirmations are short statements which help you to create a positive mental attitude, in other words – positive thinking. You can make up your own affirmations and use them to build a frame of mind which makes it possible to achieve health and happiness or whatever you want to have, be or do. You can write them down, speak them out loud or even sing them. The key to using affirmations successfully is patient repetition (ideally several times per day). Here are some simple examples:

- I am at home in my body.
- I am free to speak up for myself. I am now secure in my own expression. I communicate only with love.
- I trust in the process of life.

- My skin is perfect, healthy and clear.
- I now forgive myself (or someone else) for ...
- I am balanced in my creative flow.
- I now allow a deep, regular sleep.

Visualization

Visualization is another technique you can use to empower your mind. Like affirmations, visualization works on creating positive thought patterns to enable the changes you want in your life to occur. In visualization you use your imagination to create pictures of yourself or different parts of your body in the way that you'd like to see them.

> Imagination is more important
> than knowledge.
>
> *Albert Einstein*

Shiatsu Beauty Tips

Facial Toning

According to Oriental Medicine the Spleen function maintains the curvatures and gives support to the structures of the body. As the Spleen Ki function comes under what is termed the 'Earth Element' (*see* pages 104–5), we can appreciate the relationship of the fertility and nurturing aspects of this Element (sometimes called the 'Soil Element') and its importance to the female form. 'Earth' is considered the source of all growth and development; we can see this all around us in nature. The Spleen creates the contours and defined shapes of your body, so any 'blurring' of this muscle definition indicates impaired Spleen function. This loss of definition is most commonly seen in the face as sagging jowls, puffy eyes and loose facial skin. Try the following exercises for a fresher and more invigorated look. You'll soon notice the difference. Remember, the face is a reflection of the whole body system and so 'sagging' here indicates sagging in the internal organs.

You may do the following exercises daily in any position, but they will be most effective if you can allow yourself a bit of time and concentration. They will still be effective (but less so) if you have to do them on the way to a meeting or sitting on a bus, for example. Real change comes from within, so give yourself space to treat yourself lovingly.

Refer to fig. 7.9 for the tsubo mentioned below. Use small, spiral movements (clockwise) when focusing on specific tsubo, unless otherwise advised in the text.

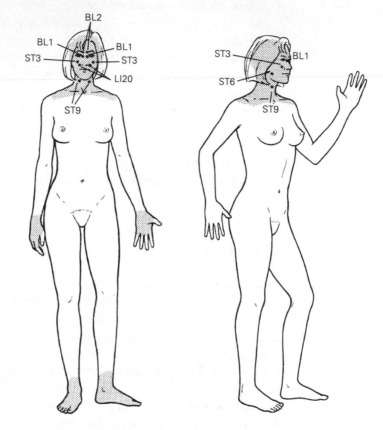

fig. 7.9 Location of ST 3, 6, 9; BL 1 and 2; LI 20

- Using the palms of your hands or your fingertips, rub your face vigorously, as if you were washing your face. Be sure to rub all over your face and include the sides of the nose, temples, upper and lower lips and jaw hinge. Rub your ears until they feel hot.
- Relax your facial muscles and open your mouth; now shake your head from side to side, so that your cheeks flap about, saying 'Aah' while you do so.
- Make a tight, puckered kiss shape with your mouth, then open the mouth as wide as possible several times. The mouth is the reflection of your digestive and reproductive systems. By improving the muscle tone of the mouth muscles you will help alleviate any weakness of the anal muscles at the other end of your digestive tract.

134

- Make your fingers into a claw shape and, making small, spiral movements of the fingertips, gently massage the forehead. Continue this movement around the temples, underneath the eyes, across the cheeks (give more concentration to the masseter 'chewing' muscles at the side of the jaw or mandible). Now focus on the chin and the upper and lower lip areas. Stimulate st 6 on both sides to activate salivation for digestion and aid Ki circulation in the hips and pelvis. Communication tension (the inability to express yourself to your own satisfaction) and sexual frustration are expressed in the 'tense jaw' look. This exercise stimulates the Ki and blood circulation to give you a more enlivened look.

- Place your thumbs under the mandible and gently press along the line of the jaw, especially under the chin and tongue root. A double chin may coincide with uterine prolapse or potential for prolapse – so take action now.

- Raise your chin, dropping the head back to stretch the muscles in the front of your neck; then tense these muscles as you lower the chin to the chest. Repeat ten times. Find and stimulate st 9, situated next to the larynx. This will help your communication generally, as well as activating the thyroid gland to function more efficiently.

- Place your index fingers at the jaw hinge next to your ears. Open and close the mouth a few times to locate the depression here. With the mouth slightly open, apply medium pressure for 30 seconds to this spot. Feel your jaw relax.

- Take hold of your ears and massage each between the thumb and index finger. Now gently pull each ear out and backwards and hold for 30 seconds. This opens the auditory canal and relieves pressure on the temporal bones (temples), which can help prevent and alleviate headaches.

- Using the pads of three fingers, gently massage the area under your eyes, to remove any congestion in the form of puffiness. Remember that this puffiness is a reflection of Deficient Kidney Ki and this needs attention through diet and exercise. Avoid stimulants such as coffee, alcohol, sugars, processed foods and recreational drugs. The Kidneys are the purifiers of the Blood and will function more effectively with fewer toxins to process and eliminate.

- Place your thumbs into the upper eye ridge and work your way from the inside (medial) to the outside (lateral). Tsubo to give attention to here are bl 1 and bl 2. bl 2 is found in the notch that you can feel in the upper orbit bone (above the eyeball). Press here, gradually applying deeper pressure, and you will feel a dull ache penetrate into your head. This is good for stimulating the brain function and relieving frontal headaches and eye ache.

- Place a thumb between the eyebrows and press firmly straight back into the forehead. 'Think' into the middle of your brain to stimulate the pituitary or 'master' gland of the endocrine system. This helps with hormonal regulation.
- For clearing the sinuses and aiding digestive functions, apply pressure to ST 3 and LI 20.
- Stick your tongue out as far as possible and say 'Aah' loudly, as if in the middle of a frustrating argument. Express yourself – you'll enjoy it.

Improve your Hair Quality

Your hair can act as an accurate indicator of your general health and, in particular, the health of your Kidney function. Thick, vibrant hair bouncing with life is a positive sign. Have you noticed how your hair lacks lustre when you are tired, stressed or otherwise ill? As mentioned in Chapter 5, Kidney Jing relates to the development of the body tissue of bone, teeth, finger nails and head hair. Part of the ageing process involves the depletion of your Kidney Jing and, therefore, the ageing of the tissue it controls. If your are suffering from excess hair loss, or your hair lacks lustre and body, you need to pay attention to enhancing your Kidney health. Stress plays a major role in reducing the effective flow of blood to the scalp and 'tires' the Kidney function. Try the following to help yourself:

- You may use a 'hand claw' technique to massage the whole scalp for 2–3 minutes daily. This involves making a hand shape like a bear's claw with rigid finger tips to contact the scalp.
- Gently pull the hair roots all over the head to stimulate the hair follicles.
- Tapping over the scalp area with lightly clenched fists helps to stimulate blood circulation and awakens the brain.
- Stimulate the following tsubo: GV 20, GV 16, GV 4, BL 23, LI 4, KID 1 and SP 6 to boost your Kidney function and for the general control of stress.
- Doing shoulder stands or hanging your torso over the end of your bed for 5–6 minutes daily will improve the blood circulation to the scalp.

The Body Scrub
This is an invigorating technique to improve the blood circulation to the skin generally and to the peripheries in particular. If an area of skin is discoloured, puffy, excessively dry or oily, try the body scrub. It is also useful as a preventative measure against the common cold, as it activates the better adaptation of your skin pores, which form part of the body's defence system. Pores that do not respond to environmental changes and remain too open will allow the external pathogens to breach your defence system governed by your Wei Ki.

Use a loufa, massage mitt, rough face flannel or towel – either wet or dry. Rub your skin vigorously until the area becomes reddened, which indicates blood coming to the surface. Cover your whole body and give particular attention to your hands, wrists, feet, ankles, buttocks, loins and abdomen. This will assist in the elimination of toxins and dead skin cells, as well as invigorating your internal membranes (also skin), which are continuous with the external skin. Your skin health is regulated primarily by the Lung Ki. Give yourself a body scrub daily and notice your improved circulation next winter.

Your Posture
Your posture is a reflection of your physical health and vitality, as well as your emotional state. Be conscious of maintaining an upright posture and avoid slumping when sitting or standing.

Physically, if your intestines are sluggish and/or emotionally, you have poor self-esteem, your posture might tend to slump forwards. This will cause a bent and stressed spine and bent internal organs. Poor posture will eventually chronically shorten and weaken your postural muscles, leading to compression of the organs and reducing the proper functioning of each organ.

Some tips for improving your posture:

- Sit in chairs that support your lower back properly.
- Place a pillow or folded hand towel under your buttocks, to raise your pelvis above the level of your knees. You can also do this in your car.
- Lift the *back* of your head towards the ceiling, as if you were being suspended by a piece of string. Mildly pull your chin towards your chest for this technique.
- Open up your chest area so that the shoulders do not collapse forwards, inhibiting your lung expansion and air intake.

- Be aware of your body being held in tension – relax your buttocks and your shoulders, as we commonly tense these unnecessarily.

Are You Overweight or Underweight?

Overweight   Being overweight or underweight may have several ramifications for your health. Firstly, whenever there is *excess* fatty tissue, which means that you are overweight, there is a toxin build-up in the body tissue. Toxins remaining in your system poison your blood and manifest themselves as a whole range of symptoms, from headaches to ovarian cysts. The extra weight means that your heart has to work harder to maintain circulation to a greater amount of tissue and so burdens all your body's homeostatic functions. Secondly, the added weight directly affects and stresses your weight-bearing joints of the legs, pelvis and spine, causing inhibited nervous system communication to your organs and endocrine (hormonal) glands.

In order to reduce weight, which may act as a physical 'buffer' of layers to protect you emotionally, you should consider several things. Firstly, do you really want to lose weight? Secondly, how can you successfully lose weight without losing your enjoyment of life and food? Thirdly, are there any 'points that I can press' to help me lose weight? Fortunately, the answer to this last question is yes, but unless you have answered the first question positively, your chances of success are limited.

You need to consider reducing your fatty acid intake – that is, animal foods including dairy products such as milk and cheese. Eat organic, whole-grain bread and only in moderation and reduce the amount of biscuits you eat, as in excess these can actually clog your bowels. Increase your intake of whole cereal grains such as brown rice, couscous and wheat pasta to strengthen the bowel, and eat more fresh fruit and vegetables, although we suggest that fruit should always be eaten as a separate course and not included with breakfast cereals or as a part of a meal.

Your next consideration is exercise. Gentle aerobic exercise to increase your intake of Air Ki and improve the strength of the lung and heart will assist in the dissolving and elimination of the stagnant Blood (fatty tissue and toxins). Regularly practise the basic exercises outlined in this book, combined with frequent gentle walking, swimming, running, cycling or aerobic exercises. If possible, talk to a physical education trainer to get some advice as to which exercise would suit you best.

Self-treatment involves reducing the excess water in your system, tonifying the strength of your Stomach and Lung Ki to help improve the production of Grain Ki (Nutritive Ki) and Air Ki, and the reduction of any mucus deposits in the system (*see* the Physiological Sink in Chapter 8).

To tonify the Stomach and Lung energies, treat ST 25 and 36, LU 7 and 1, LI 4 and SP 6. To remove the excess water, supplement the above treatment with the addition of CV 9, SP 9, BL 23 and BL 54. Dissolving mucus requires the type of exercise described above, plus the pelvic floor exercises described in Chapter 8 in Strengthening your Ovarian Palace. Drinking camomile tea and eating 'dissolving' foods such as shitake mushrooms, radish and pickled vegetables will also help with this.

Underweight — Being underweight may also be a stress factor for consideration, particularly in cases of infertility. People who sporadically attempt severe diets combined with excess amounts of exercise and even excess sex will injure their Kidney Yin (the stored energy of the kidneys). Heavily restrictive diets and crash diets have been found to be more injurious than beneficial, and can even cause serious problems such as heart attack.[3] Weight is a balance between energy intake, the storage (Grain/Nutritive Ki stored as Yin) of water and glycogen and the expenditure of energy (Yang activity). If your lifestyle is such that you expend more energy than you take in, then you will not only lose fat tissue but also dip into your reserves and so weaken your Yin. This leads to a drying-out of the body, including the mucus and other lubricants necessary for internal organ functioning – a Yin Deficiency condition.

This dryness and lack of muscle fuel lead to lethargy and weaken your Wei Ki, which leaves you more susceptible to External pathogens. Irritations and inflammations in the pelvic organs and the deficiency of water in the system may lead to constipation (a dry disorder), or Heat in the Blood causing excessive vaginal bleeding. It can also result in the formation of scar tissue in your Fallopian tubes, ovaries or fimbriae, causing infertility.

This is therefore a condition of Dryness with Deficient Kidney Yin (water) and Excess Liver Yang (heat and activity). Treat KID 1 and 10, BL 23, GB 25, and SP 6 to tonify the Kidney Yin; LIV2 and 3 to control and relax the Liver Yang; CV 6 and 7, and GV 4 to enhance the pelvic organ function. Avoid excessive cardiovascular exercise and introduce more Do-In-style exercise to calm the nervous system and move the Ki. Drink at least two litres (three and a half pints) of water daily and avoid dry saunas (steam rooms are fine as they are moist). Do not have penetrative sex during menstruation and ideally reduce the amount of penetrative sex generally for two or three months, as this taxes the Kidney Yin. Eat Kidney Yin-restorative foods like aduki beans, black beans, oysters, squid, raspberries and strawberries.

chapter 8

Shiatsu for Sexuality and Sensuality

There is a general conception of shiatsu as a therapeutic treatment for alleviating aches and pains and improving different body functions. This is of course true, for shiatsu is great for health management on both a physical and mental level. It is also true, however, that a good state of psycho-emotional health should bring physical benefits to more than just your muscles – and it does. Because you are relaxing and enhancing your nervous system through shiatsu, you will find that you become more 'focused', with faster reactions both mentally and physically. You will also feel your vitality improve and find that life seems more enjoyable and less stressful. You will notice that your appetite for food feels more active and that your 'appetite for life', particularly your sexual appetite, is awakening with a smile.

The interaction we have with others on an everyday basis is on a fundamental sexual communication level. This does not mean that everyone you meet has sex on their mind – only a few of them! What is does mean, however, is that natural attraction and the way you communicate with others comes from your 'appetite for life' – that is, an interest in people at all levels, which does include both physical and mental 'contact'. It's that 'spark' which makes the difference between a close friend and an acquaintance.

We have already talked about the Kidney energy as the basis for our existence, having stored the Jing or constitutional strength. This is your 'life spark', the fire of your passion for life. The Kidney Fire is the motivating force behind your sexual libido, as it warms the Ki and makes it more active. Your sexual libido is a hot-natured manifestation, which affects both your mind and body. It can also be expressed in your passion for arguing, laughing, dancing, shouting and joyful mischievousness. These are all signs of enjoying life and are often suppressed by education and society's inhibitions. This passion is the 'fire in your belly' and it, too, needs attention and nurturing to keep the flames alight.

Sex and Stress Don't Mix

Stress is a real 'turn off' to most of your enjoyable body functions. Anxiety about life in general or specific issues will injure your Spleen Yin. How you see yourself and your feelings of self-assuredness and self-empowerment reside in the Spleen – so think 'calm'. Remember, you have a *choice* to be stressed or not to be stressed. Take control and empower yourself!

When you are stressed, your Liver Ki (usually responsible for the free flow of Ki in your body) becomes stagnant. You too become stagnant, without vitality and the flow of your passion for life. When the Liver and Spleen are battling it out for control, this exhausts your Kidney Ki and it is often your libido that suffers. Thinking too much means that energy is distracted into your head and so does not go to the Lower Burner (abdomen) where it is needed. The Lower Burner cools and becomes dormant and you may feel 'distant' and less outwardly expressive. This is hardly a good basis for a happy sexual relationship.

How to Help your Sexual Enjoyment

To increase your sexual pleasure perform the Do-In exercises in Chapter 7 regularly (to balance your meridian system), combined with the relaxation meditation techniques to help relieve stress and, as often as possible, get your partner to give you some shiatsu as described in Chapter 4. Unfortunately, there are no 'magic points' to make you or your partner instantly amorous, but here are some tips to help you enjoy yourselves more.

The first guideline is to think about the shiatsu in a different way – that is, as *Tantric* shiatsu and not the type you usually receive from a professional shiatsu therapist. Allow it to feel like foreplay and give and receive with gentle and loving sensuality. Try it without clothes for the best results.

142

- Rub your hands together vigorously, to give greater sensitivity and sensuality to them.
- Gently and rhythmically rock your partner all over, starting at the shoulders and moving down to the feet. This relaxes the nervous system.
- Get as close to your partner as is comfortable and try to be sensual in all the movements you make. For example, if you are working on your partner's back, squat over their buttocks with your thighs across the backs of their thighs.
- Do the general back treatment movements from Chapter 4, adding long, gliding strokes and gentle, rubbing finger caresses along the spine and back muscles. This will help any tension to melt away and the nervous system to relax and so heighten your partner's physical sensitivity.
- Give particular attention to the lower back muscles and the buttocks. Use your forearms like rolling pins and make sweeping movements across their buttocks. If you can relax the buttocks, the pelvis Ki will flow more freely.
- Make small, spiral movements in a clockwise direction at the following points to build the Fire in their Lower Burner and genitals: BL 23 in the mid-lumbar area; the indentations in the sacrum (BL 31–4); at the base of the sacrum (GV 2); in the middle of the perineum between the genitals and the anus (CV 1).
- With one hand on top of the other, make circular movements (clockwise) over your partner's abdomen, gently using your fingertips to massage away any tight areas.
- Whenever 'the moment' arises, move from these sensual massage movements to other foreplay. Enjoy!

The Female Reproductive System
Anatomy
Your reproductive organs are part of the genitourinary system as follows:

Primary Organs:	ovaries
Secondary Organs:	vagina, cervix, Fallopian tubes, uterus

The urinary system comprises the kidneys, ureters, bladder and urethra.

fig. 8.1 The female
reproductive system
with organ locations

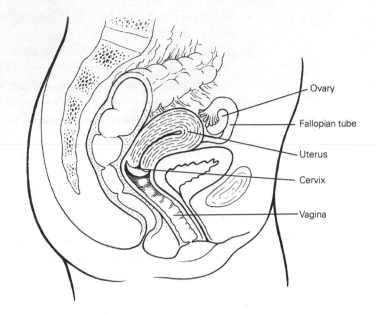

Ovary

Fallopian tube

Uterus

Cervix

Vagina

Yin/Yang Energetics

By virtue of the position of these organs in the body, they are much affected by gravity. From the mouth, the process of digestion moves downwards
through the digestive system (with the separation of the 'pure' from the
'impure'), through the excretory system, to be expelled in the form of waste
by-products: faeces and urine (the 'impure') as well as menstrual blood.

A woman's reproductive organs are influenced predominately by Yin
energy. They are thus located deeper or more internally and are more dense
in structure, especially the primary organs, the ovaries. By comparison, a
man's primary organs of reproduction have more of a Yang influence and
are located externally, especially the primary organs of the testes. They
also have a less dense structure. The actual function of these organs is
affected by their energetic nature – that is, the process of ejaculation is a
more upwards and active Yang manifestation; the movement of the ovum
is a slower and downwards Yin manifestation. When these Ki-charged cells
meet, a Yin/Yang balance is created – a cosmic explosion when the prenatal *Yuan Ki* (Original Ki) is formed and conception occurs.

The Physiological 'Sink'

The reproductive organs in the average woman tend to act like a physiological 'sink' – that is, the excess waste products of the body that are unsuc-
cessfully excreted deposit in this area. The circulation of Ki and Blood

through the pelvic viscera is controlled by the hara energy, muscular movement and the pelvic diaphragm (urogenital diaphragm). Energetically, this is the home of the Liver Ki circulation and the Lower Burner of the Three Burners – energy confluence areas which have a controlling, regulating and warming function in relation to their surrounding organs. This Lower Burner area is situated between the navel and the pubis. In the Orient this area is called the *Ovarian Palace*; in the male the same area is called the *Sperm Palace*.

Due to our predominately sedentary lifestyles, the muscles in these areas may become flaccid, the diaphragm restricted and, as a result of this, the Ki flow becomes sluggish and stagnant. Poor Liver patency results in stagnant Ki (the Ki 'draws' the Blood) and therefore stagnant Blood. There is commonly a *Cold* syndrome apparent, which can result in an aversion to cold, bladder chills, copious urinations, weak pelvic muscles (which may eventually manifest themselves as a prolapse), and coldness and pain in the lower abdomen. *Damp*, another External influence, accumulates due to living in cold and damp environments, taking in excess salt and dairy products, or lack of exercise and poor eating habits. The symptoms of this condition may be physical fatigue, poor appetite, heavy limbs, abdominal bloating, scanty urinations, swelling in the ankles and hands, and a thick greasy coating on the tongue. If chronic low-level inflammation and irritation such as a thrush condition are experienced, a *Heat* pattern is prevalent. The symptoms for this might include fever, aversion to heat, desire for cold foods and drink, a flushed complexion, dark urine, sharp abdominal pains, blood or mucus in the stools, or burning sensations when either urinating or defecating. There may also be redness around the genitals or general irritation in this area.

Like a sink, the more water containing waste matter placed there and left undisturbed, the greater the accumulation and hardening effect of the sediment materials. This manifests itself as congestion as the waste settles to the bottom. Lack of movement allows continued accumulation, which may take the form of obstructions such as cysts and tumours (Blood stagnation). The pelvic viscera also includes organs of elimination, specifically the small and large bowel and the urinary bladder, all aiding in the elimination of the 'impure' Essence refined from your food and drink (Grain Ki or Gu Ki).

Exercise and improved diet are obvious methods of remedying this situation. Remove the toxins in your diet as these worsen the congestion; add in foods that help dissolve the congestion, such as mustard seed, radish and shitake mushrooms; and introduce some exercise to circulate the Ki and

Blood. These measures will result in improved blood and lymph flow, greater absorption and excretion potential in the bowel, and thus the expelling of the waste remaining in the pelvic viscera.

Strengthening your Ovarian Palace

The following simple, yet very effective, exercises will improve the blood and Ki circulation in this area and strengthen the pelvic floor muscles. For purpose of these exercises, consider these muscles as having a front (anterior) area influencing mostly the vagina, uterus, Fallopian tubes, ovaries and bladder; and a rear (posterior) section influencing the colon, bladder and uterus (*see* fig. 8.2). The musculature of your pelvis creates a suspension for the uterus, attached to the internal 'bowl' of the pelvis by muscle and fascia. This is why poor posture and the subsequent distortion of the pelvic girdle bones may affect the functioning of your reproductive organs. Create a routine for doing these exercises daily – before going to bed or upon awakening, for example – and then whenever you remember throughout the day.

fig. 8.2 The pelvic bowl showing the two (anterior and posterior) triangles of muscular influence of the vagina and anus

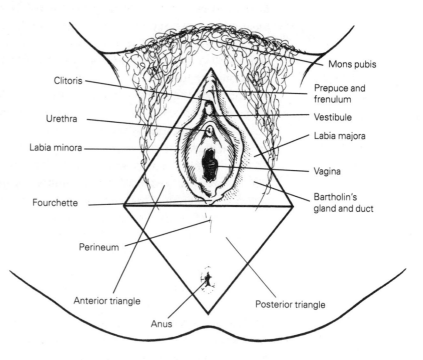

Mons pubis

Clitoris

Prepuce and frenulum

Urethra

Vestibule

Labia majora

Labia minora

Vagina

Bartholin's gland and duct

Fourchette

Perineum

Anterior triangle

Posterior triangle

Anus

Shiatsu for Sexuality and Sensuality

Exercise One   This exercise strengthens your Liver meridian and Central Channel, both of which pass through the vagina, cervix and uterus. The Chinese referred to this area as the 'Gate of Life' from which new life develops.

1) Sit comfortably in a chair, on the floor or even lie down.
2) Breathe into your hara (abdomen) by expanding your abdominal muscles, like a balloon filling, as you breathe in. On the exhalation, contract your abdominal muscles to flatten your abdomen. Repeat three times for relaxation.
3) On your next inhalation, expand your muscles while 'pushing down' into your genitals – you will feel your pelvic floor respond. Pull up on the pelvic floor as you exhale. Repeat three times.
4) Focus into your vagina muscles and squeeze; lift and release these muscles ten times in quick succession. Try another ten repetitions until you feel warmth in your vagina – this indicates improved blood flow. You may have difficulty 'contacting' your internal muscles for the first few attempts, but this will change with practice.
5) As you become experienced with this exercise, you can 'think' into your vagina as you pull upwards and draw the Ki into your uterus, Fallopian tubes and ovaries. Feel a glowing warmth spread throughout the pelvis.

Exercise Two   Another useful exercise relates to your urinations, as your urethra and bladder are part of the genitourinary system. The exercise involves controlling the urination flow:

- Start your urination flow, allow about one third of your waters to pass and then squeeze your vaginal pelvic floor muscles until the flow stops for a moment. Resume your flow again.
- Repeat two or three times with each urination. With practice you will be able to completely stop your flow at will – an indication of improved muscle tonus.
- Please note that it is harmful to 'hold off' urinating for any length of time, as this strains the bladder. Go to the toilet as soon as possible when you feel the urge to urinate.

These exercises will not only help to improve your pelvic floor muscles for the regulation of menstruation and better elimination, but also have the added benefit of allowing for more enjoyable sex, as you will have greater control of your vaginal muscles and may experience an enhanced intensity in your orgasm.

chapter 9

Shiatsu for Pregnancy and Childbirth

Shiatsu and the Nature of Pregnancy

> Treating a disease after it has arisen,
> is the lowest level of healthcare and treatment.
>
> *The Nei Ching*

Pregnancy is a very natural condition and should not be seen as a disease. However, it will put great demands upon your physical body and spirit. *Preparing* yourself for conceiving, as soon as you decide you want children, is therefore recommended. A combination of diet adjustments, exercises and relaxation should all feature in your preparation, as the ease of your pregnancy and birth will depend to a great extent on your general health and well-being at the time.

The Physical and Metaphysical Development of a Foetus

> In the first month, it is a pulp
> In the second month, it is a ball
> In the third month, it is a foetus
> In the fourth month, there is flesh

> In the fifth month, there are muscles
> In the sixth month, there are bones
> In the seventh month, the man is formed
> In the eight month, it moves
> In the ninth month, it becomes impatient
> In the tenth month, it sees the day.
>
> *Huainanzi, second century* BC

Oriental philosophy draws a parallel between life in the womb and the 2.8 billion years of the evolution of life on earth as it developed in the 'Water Phase'. This amphibian period is thought to correspond to 280 days of pregnancy, in which the foetus evolves from a single cell to a multicellular being: 'One grain, ten thousand grains', as the Chinese would say. So from this we can deduce that ten million years of evolution is occurring for every day of pregnancy.

Every day of pregnancy helps for a more 'developed' being in the physical and metaphysical realms. At birth, the following energies initiate a life pattern in the 'Land Phase': the *Lung* energy is responsible for the child breathing independently air and not liquid; the *Triple Heater* has to 'spark' into life to heat the child outside of the warm, water state; the *Heart Protector* activates for emotional/spiritual protection outside the secure womb. The providing of a happy and secure environment for the foetus 'in embryo' and subsequently for entry into the Land Phase needs to be the underlying principle for parental care and shiatsu assistance.

The Energy Connection between Mother and Child

In Japan they consider *Tai Kyo* (embryo education) to be very important for the development of the foetus. In the East it is traditionally thought that one third of our ultimate social, physical and mental functioning is already determined by our experiences in the womb. Pregnant women in Japan, therefore, are encouraged to listen to calming music and to avoid loud or frightening sounds, for example. Water is a very good conductor of sound and the foetus in its watery environment is sensitive to auditory stimulation from the outside world, as well as the sounds from the mother's own internal organs. The mother's heartbeat will be very calming for the foetus.

Some research shows that the foetus is most comfortable when the mother is moving slowly, such as during steady walking or crawling. This is probably because such movements give the foetus the effect of being rocked. Crawling and being down on all fours also creates a bit more space for the foetus in the womb.

The foetus is provided with continuous tactile stimulation from the internal environment through the amniotic fluid (the clear fluid surrounding the foetus in the uterus) and the walls of the sac. Shiatsu and massage, applied from the outside, will give the foetus a similar experience. The external touch sends energy vibrations inwards, which then create movements internally. So here is an excellent opportunity to start giving your baby appropriate stimulation even before birth.

Early Indications of Pregnancy

Before the use of microscopic investigations, the Chinese believed that conception occurred as a result of the mixing of the women's 'red' Essence, the menstrual blood, with the male 'white' essence, the sperm. Today, however, we know that conception occurs in the Fallopian tube within 60 minutes of ejaculation. Sperm passes through the acidic medium of the uterus to the more alkaline Fallopian tube. Once the ovum has been fertilized, its magnetic charge changes and no longer attracts more sperm. After a day or two the fertilized ovum journeys to the uterus for implantation and sustenance by blood in the 'Blood Chamber'.

A pregnant woman may experience all or some of the following: amenorrhoea; breast swelling; sickness; fatigue (progesterone in the bloodstream acts as a tranquillizer); 'blossoming'; colour change (facial hue); change in metabolic rate; revulsion at fatty, oily food (all relate to Liver function); sweet cravings (Spleen function); increase in frequency of passing urine; swelling or weight gain. She may also know intuitively that she is pregnant from the moment of conception.

Energetic Changes during Pregnancy

The 'vital' organs of a pregnant woman will have to cope with the support and maintenance of two 'beings' right from the moment of conception. For this reason, profound changes take place in the Zang organs of the mother. The foetal *Original* or *Yuan Ki*, initiated at the moment of the polarity charge between ovum and sperm, sustains the embryo until the placenta develops. From the cosmic 'charge' of the Yin/Yang attraction there appears a preponderance of Blood and Ki. The Blood congeals as the Heart sends the Blood to nourish the embryo in the womb. The foetus will then exist off the mother's *Blood* – that is, the energy created by the Liquid essence of her Spleen, the Original and Acquired Ki of her Kidney energy and the circulation and sustenance of the Heart Yang and Ki from the Lungs. The Blood will be the nourishment for her child. The Fire of conception continues to ensure that the Blood nurtures them both.

The function of the Spleen is challenged as the increase of Damp prevails to form the amniotic fluid to nourish and protect the embryo. The Spleen energy will become Deficient and the Liver Ki will maintain the patency of the flow of the energy in the womb, and indeed in both the mother and foetus. The Liver energy will become Excess. Because the mother is supplying her Yuan Ki and the Kidney Yin and Kidney Yang, her Kidney energy will become Deficient. All these symptoms are considered symptoms of a single causation – that is, pregnancy – and are all perfectly normal.

How Shiatsu Can Help during Pregnancy

In the Orient, pregnancy is regarded as spiritual practice. It is felt that a pregnant woman should spend as much of her time as possible 'in prayer and contemplation'. She is recommended to surround herself both physically and emotionally with things that are pleasant and comforting, and to focus on the moral and mental education of the foetus through spiritual practice.

Though it is impossible for a pregnant woman to stay serene all the time, it is advisable to prevent stress and anxiety from reaching levels that might adversely affect her mental state of mind and negatively affect her baby. Shiatsu is a wonderful way of getting in touch with the positive, natural changes that will occur during pregnancy. It gives an increased awareness of the body, both physically and emotionally, and offers a great opportunity to tune in to the unborn baby. We will now look at each stage of pregnancy, with recommendations for exercises and diet where appropriate, before going on to look at the most common ailments suffered during pregnancy and the relevant self-treatment approach.

First Trimester: 0–12 weeks

Your pregnancy can be divided into three parts or trimesters, according to the development of the foetus. You cannot see your baby growing inside you, but there are some incredible changes taking place internally. During the first trimester all systems of the foetus are developing, with many organs more or less complete. According to Oriental Medicine, the Kidney is the first organ to develop. In fact, the foetus is regarded as a big Kidney from which all the other organs later emerge and develop individually.

By the end of the first trimester, the nerves and muscles of the foetus are working and reflexes are establishing. Even if you cannot feel any movements yet, your baby can spontaneously move at this stage. Due to all this internal activity in the development of the foetus, the focus during the first three months of pregnancy should be on support and nurturing and not so much interference from the outside. Allow yourself and your body to tune in to the internal changes and try to create some time for relaxation. Exercise is important and you can focus on Do-In exercises in combination with meridian stretching exercises (*see* Chapter 7). Walking and swimming will also be good. A general soothing and calming treatment from a friend or your partner will also be very beneficial, but avoid any deeper pressure, any strong stretches or strong pressure below the pelvis (*see* Contraindications on pages 155–6).

Common complaints during the first trimester are general fatigue and tiredness, morning sickness and breast tenderness. Refer to pages 156–65 for your treatment approach.

Second Trimester: 13–27 weeks
After the first three months, the pregnancy is usually more stable. This is a period of rapid growth when you will become noticeably pregnant. You will be able to feel foetal movements and your baby will be starting to look like a real person as well as to behave like one.

Treat any specific conditions as they arise, but you should still avoid any strong pressure below the pelvis and any strong stretches. Try to keep up the exercise programme mentioned earlier, and include the exercises described on pages 166–71. These will promote deeper breathing, increase the flexibility of the pelvic muscles and ligaments, strengthen your abdominal muscles and generally prepare you for the delivery of your baby. You could also attend yoga classes for pregnant women, as a useful preparation for the birth.

Hopefully any morning sickness will have eased off by now and you can nourish yourself and your baby through a well-balanced diet. Since the foetus is feeding off your Blood, it is important to include food in your diet which will promote Blood production. Fresh vegetables are essential, in particular dark green, leafy vegetables. Yellow vegetables, such as carrots and winter squash, are also good. Most beans and several seafoods will strengthen the Blood, and small amounts of animal protein, especially in soups and broths, will also be beneficial. Try to eat warming, cooked food and less cold, raw food. Your food should be fresh and freshly prepared to ensure a good quality of Ki, as Ki builds the Blood.

Third Trimester: 28–40 weeks

During the third trimester, your baby elongates and starts to accumulate fat. The baby is now much stronger and the movements in the womb can be quite vigorous and clear. Towards the end of the third trimester the baby gains 28 grams (1 ounce) per day, fills your uterus and settles into the position for birth, with the head descending into the pelvis. Yes, that is why you feel you need to go to the toilet constantly.

Due to the extra weight from the growing foetus, together with the softening of the pelvic region, back pain is a very common complaint during this time. To ease off the pain, get your partner to apply pressure to the sacrum area using their thumbs. This can be done in side position or kneeling (*see* Chapter 4). Gentle rubbing of the area will also be beneficial. To relieve back pain on your own:

- Lie down on your back, bringing the knees up towards your chest allowing space for your belly. Hold on to your knees and feel the sacrum against the floor. Slowly make circular movements with your knees and feel your sacrum and lower back being massaged against the floor.
- Rock back and forth, still with your hand around your knees. Roll up to squatting position, feet apart and the buttocks off the floor.

You might feel compression of the ribs as the uterus rises and/or due to the high position of the baby's head before it drops down in the pelvic cavity prior to birth. Some women suffer discomfort from pressure on the diaphragm and a shortness of breath. To alleviate these conditions, prop yourself up with cushions into a half-lying position. For extra support, place a rolled-up towel underneath your upper back – this will create expansion of the chest. Try the following breathing exercise:

- Close your eyes and bring your awareness to your breathing. Become aware of the breath entering into your body through your nose and allow yourself to relax with each breath. Focus on your solar plexus area and feel the Ki from your breath reaching this space of your body. Use your breath and Ki to gently relax this area, slowly allowing it to open up and expand. Feel the chest expanding as you breathe in and feel the breath passing through the solar plexus area down to your belly.
- Give yourself 10–15 minutes to practise this exercise. When in discomfort, get your partner to support the release of your diaphragm by

placing one hand underneath your back at the area opposite the solar plexus, and the other hand on top covering the area just below the sternum (solar plexus area – *see* fig. 9.1). You will gradually feel the tension go and the muscles relax and it will feel easier to breathe afterwards.

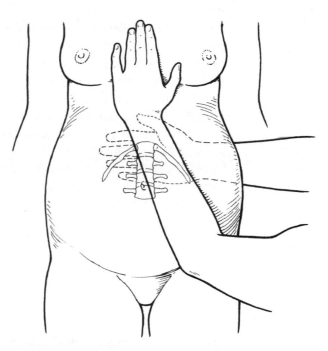

fig. 9.1
Diaphragm release

Dos and Don'ts during Pregnancy (Contraindications)

Some of the tsubo or acupressure points we use in shiatsu treatments are considered contraindicated during pregnancy. These points all have an eliminating quality and stimulating them will have a releasing action on the uterus containing the foetus. (As this is precisely what you want to achieve during delivery, you will find that some of these contraindicated points are recommended in the section about childbirth.)

The following points should be avoided during your pregnancy, unless treating specific problems:

- 'Shoulder Well', GB 21
- 'Adjoining Valleys,' LI 4
- 'Arm Three Mile', LI 10 (cautionary point only)
- 'Three Yin Junction', SP 6
- 'Foot Three Miles', ST 36

155

- 'Great Thoroughfare', LIV 3
- 'Gushing Spring', KID 1

Self-Treatments for Common Ailments
Anaemia
This is a Blood Deficiency syndrome showing itself in symptoms such as: a pallid complexion, pale lips and eyelids, pale fingernails, a lack of vitality, breathlessness, palpitations, a sore tongue (inflamed) and headaches. If the Blood is Deficient you need to tonify it to alleviate your anaemic condition. The best way to do this is through a healthy diet rich in green vegetables and whole grains (*see* the recommendations under Second Trimester, page 153). Drink mugwort tea (available from Chinese food and herb shops) or *Ume-sho-bancha* daily – *bancha* twig tea with three drops of soy sauce and an *Umeboshi* plum, the Japanese sour plum (you can find them in Japanese food shops and some health-food stores). Seaweed will also be very beneficial and you can try toasted *Nori* sheets as a complement to your diet (buy them from Japanese food and some health-food shops). As an extra supplement, buy Floradex herbal tonic from your nearest health-food store.

Treatment   Apply pressure to following tsubo: SP 6 and 10, TB 6 and GV 22 (*see* fig. 9.2).

Please note for reference to all illustrations:
All tsubo are bilaterally located on the body unless found on the midline. Shaded areas indicate where to give general shiatsu treatment.

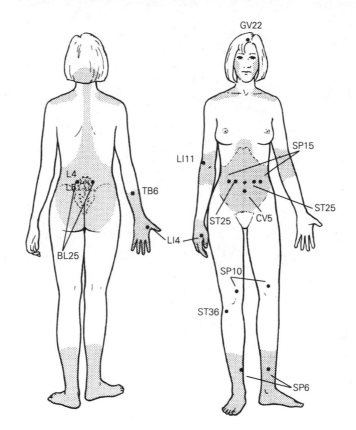

fig. 9.2 Anaemia/
constipation: point
location chart

Breast Tenderness
Enlarged, tender breasts are one of the first signs of pregnancy.

Treatment For relief, gently massage your breast with circular movements and apply
gentle pressure to the following points using your palms or fingers: ST 13
and 16, and KID 22 (*see* fig. 9.3). Treat the Stomach meridian in your legs as
described under Heartburn on page 160.

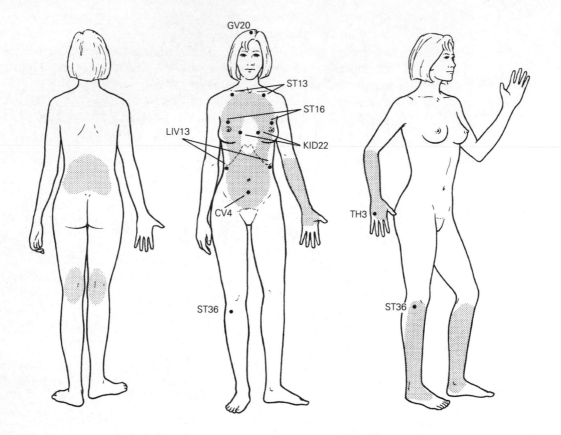

fig. 9.3 Breast
tenderness/low energy:
point location chart

Breech Position
A breech baby will sit in the uterus with the head up and bottom down.
Most babies are in this position at some time during the pregnancy, but
usually they turn upside down (cephalic position) of their own accord.

Treatment   If you discover that your baby is in breech position after the 32nd week, try
to encourage your baby to turn itself using the following exercise:

- Lie on the floor with your hips raised on a few pillows and your head and shoulders on the floor. Make an 'energy contact' with your baby, using the visualization techniques described in Chapter 7 – tune in to the movements of your baby. Visualize the baby turning around into a correct position.
- Give yourself 10–15 minutes in this position, two or three times every day, and encourage the baby to move with the head into the pelvis. Take advantage of this time to relax, perhaps with the help of some music.

You can also stimulate the point on the outer edge of your little toes (BL 67), using your finger, thumb or nail. A shiatsu practitioner would apply moxibustion to this point in the last three weeks of pregnancy – a very successful method of treatment. Alternatively, you could use a cigarette instead of the herb stick to help the baby move, although a cigarette is not as strong. Hold it over BL 67 (half a centimetre from the skin) until the skin becomes hot; repeat six times, two or three times per day, until the baby moves. The homoeopathic remedy *Pulsatilla* will also be beneficial, as it too has a reputation for turning breech babies.

Constipation
Progesterone causes a relaxation of the muscles of your intestines during pregnancy and this slows down your bowel movements, which can result in constipation. This is more harmful than you might think, as it leads to toxins spreading throughout your body. To help prevent this, exercise daily and eat a diet rich in whole grains and fibre foods, including fruit and vegetables. (*See also* page 153.)

Treatment   Regular, full shiatsu treatments will be very beneficial. Get your partner to give you some Kenbiki massage down your back, as explained in Chapter 3 and apply pressure to the following tsubo: ST 25 and 36, SP15, BL 25, CV 5, LI 4 and LI 11 (*see* fig. 9.2).

Heartburn

This is really a sensation that comes from your stomach. The valve at the entrance to your stomach organ relaxes in pregnancy, allowing small amounts of acid to get into the oesophagus. This gives a burning sensation behind the breastbone, which is why we call it 'heartburn'. To prevent this condition, avoid any food that tends to bring it on and do not lie down within two hours of eating. Remember to chew well and eat small meals throughout the day.

Treatment Release the diaphragm as described earlier in this chapter (*see* under Third Trimester, pages 154–5) and give shiatsu to the front of your legs, along the Stomach meridian. Sit on the floor with one foot beneath you, using your elbow or thumb (*see* fig. 9.4) to apply pressure from the hip down to the knee. Apply pressure to the following tsubo: ST 25, CV 12 and 14, LI 4 and BL 21 (*see* fig. 9.5).

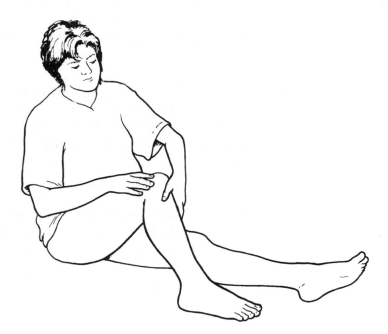

fig. 9.4 Self-treatment of
the Stomach meridian

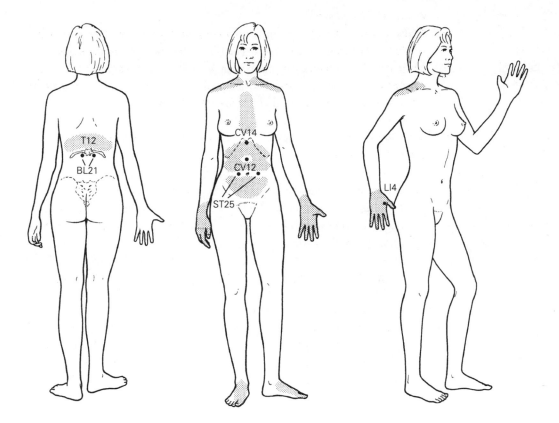

fig. 9.5 Heartburn: point location chart

Low Energy Level – Fatigue
This is a particular problem if you do not acknowledge the physical and emotional demands a pregnancy will have on your body. Make sure you take breaks during your working day and allow time for relaxation. These rest times will also give you an opportunity to connect with your growing baby, using visualization and/or affirmations (*see* Chapter 7).

Treatment   Apply pressure to: ST 36, LIV 13, CV 4, TB 3 and GV 20 (*see* fig. 9.3).

Shiatsu for Women

Morning Sickness
Many women suffer from nausea or morning sickness, which is usually caused by hormonal changes. It is still not clear why it affects some women and not others, although your diet before conception will have an influence. A diet low in vitamins, carbohydrates and minerals will be predisposing. Tiredness will also contribute negatively.

Treatment In Oriental Medicine we distinguish between three different kinds of morning sickness:

1)   Rotten and muddy Ki rebelling – *the symptoms here will include belching, abdominal swelling, congested lungs, depression and hiccoughs. Clear the Stomach energy by applying pressure to HG 6, ST 36 and 44 (see fig. 9.6).*
2)   Mucus and fluid toxin – *the vital organs are suffering from shock. Dizziness, vomiting watery liquid, a white-coated tongue, low energy and general coldness will be among the symptoms here. Treat the above plus ST 40 (see fig. 9.6).*
3)   Rising Fire of Liver – *Kidney energy is exhausted in the uterus, the Liver lacks Yin and dries, and this damages the Stomach Ki. Symptoms may include a bitter taste, belching, rib pain, pain in the area behind and below your lower ribs and a rapid pulse. Formula number 1 above plus apply pressure to LIV 2 and GB 34 (see fig. 9.6).*

Generally, eat dry biscuits (oatcakes or rice cakes) and drink *bancha* twig tea (available from some health-food stores and Japanese food shops). Peppermint and raspberry leaf tea are classical remedies for prenatal nausea. Avoid the intake of caffeine and alcohol and try the old Oriental remedy of eating *Umeboshi*. Eat small but nutritious meals during the day and chew your food thoroughly. Grapes and papaya are also well tolerated.

Oedema
Many women suffer from swollen hands and feet in late pregnancy due to an increase of the amount of fluid retained (a result of the pressure of the uterus on the blood vessels that return blood to the heart from the lower parts of the body). Symptoms of oedema may include swelling of the four limbs, the face, eyes, groin and ankles; coldness in your abdomen; a yellow or dark skin colour; Excess chest and nasal mucus; a sticky mouth; an aversion to cold and a need for hot drinks. (*See also* page 203.)

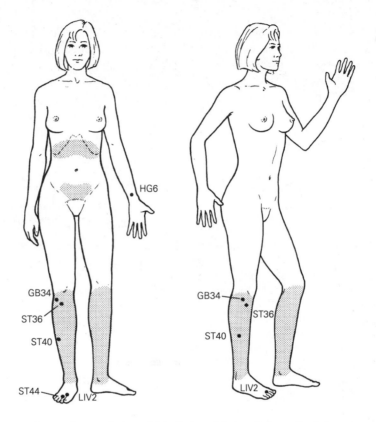

HG6

GB34
ST36
ST40
ST44 — LIV2

GB34
ST36
ST40
LIV2

fig. 9.6 Morning
sickness: point
location chart

According to Oriental Medicine this is a Spleen Deficiency condition
with Blood stagnation in the hara. Make yourself a daikon drink – squeeze
the juice from half a cup of grated daikon or radish into warm water (one
part daikon to three parts water), add several drops of soy sauce or sea salt.
Bring to the boil and simmer for 1 minute. Drink once daily for three days
maximum. This will increase sweating and urination and work as a diuret-
ic to get rid of excess fluid. Daily exercise which makes you sweat will also
help. Control your liquid intake and drink when thirsty rather than just
out of habit.

Treatment   Rest with your legs elevated daily and practise Do-In exercises on your
legs. Apply pressure to the following tsubo: ST 45, SP 9 and 10, CV 5 and
BL 20 (*see* fig. 9.7).

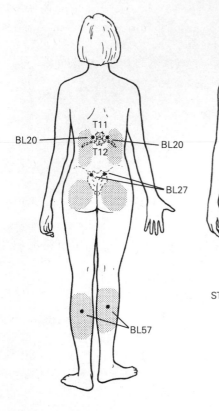
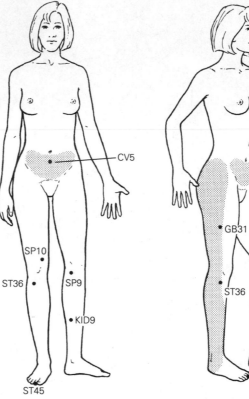

fig. 9.7 Oedema/tired
legs and leg cramps:
point location chart

Tired Legs and Leg Cramps
These are common complaints during pregnancy and may be due to poor
circulation or deficiencies in your diet (low levels of calcium in the blood).

Treatment Try any of the following:

- Use the Do-In techniques described in Chapter 7 to enhance the
  energy flow in the leg meridians.
- Rest on your back with your legs supported on a chair or cushions.
- When sitting, keep your feet higher than hip level.
- Stretch the back of your legs by standing at arm's length from a wall,
  with your hand flat against it at shoulder height and your feet directly
  under your hip joint. Bend your arms and slowly lean forwards, keeping your knees straight and your feet flat on the floor. You should feel
  the stretch down your calf muscle (*see* fig. 9.8).

164

- Sitting on the floor with your legs in front of you, press BL 54 behind your knee and, with your other hand, bring your toes and foot up towards the ceiling (*see* fig. 9.9 overleaf).
- Apply pressure to GB 31, BL 27 and 57, KID 9 and ST 36 (*see* fig. 9.7)

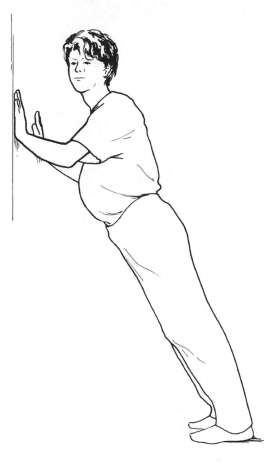

fig. 9.8 Standing stretch
of the Bladder channel

fig. 9.9
Self-treatment of BL 54

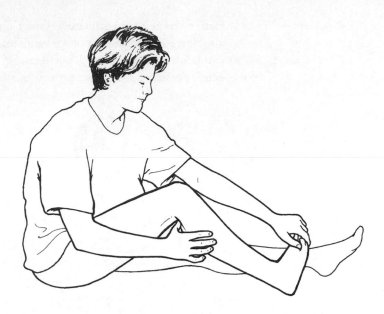

Strengthening Exercises during Pregnancy

A regular exercise programme during your pregnancy will be very beneficial for your muscles, ligaments and bony structure. The special exercises
recommended here will help in preparing your body for the process of
birth. They are designed to promote deep breathing, strengthen your muscles and increase the flexibility of your pelvic muscles and ligaments. If
you are not used to exercising, remember to start slowly with only a few
exercises, and then gradually increase the exercise time as you feel
stronger and more familiar with the different movements involved.

From an Oriental view, the rib cage is related to the pelvis. To improve
the flexibility of the pelvis, practise exercises that will open the rib cage.
Try the following two exercises:

The Bellows • Sit on the floor with your knees bent and open, with the soles of your feet together. Straighten your spine and bring your palms together in front of your chest, with the fingers pointed upwards and elbows out to the side (*see* fig. 9.10). Inhale deeply.

• As you exhale, open up your arms to the sides, with fingers still pointed upwards. Expand your rib cage as much as possible. Breathe in as you return to the starting position. Repeat at least six times.

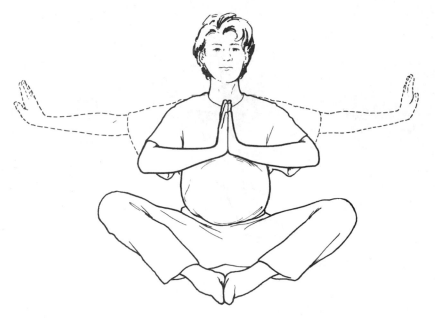

fig. 9.10 The Bellows

The Butterfly • Sit as in the previous exercise and clasp your hands around your feet. Bring your feet as close to your body as you can without slumping, and gently bounce your legs up and down. This will relax your lower abdomen, as well as working on the flexibility of your legs.

One of the most common complaints during pregnancy is back pain. The following exercise will release tension in your back and loins and also help release toxins from your digestive tract.

167

The Cat
- Get down on all fours, keeping your knees shoulder-width apart. Take a deep breath in and arch your back up towards the ceiling, like a cat, allowing your head to hang loose.
- On an exhalation, relax your back and arch your head up and back (*see* fig. 9.11). Repeat this exercise five to ten times and then come to a squatting position.

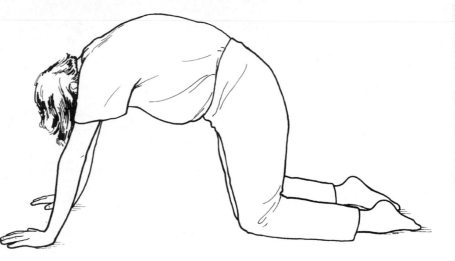

fig. 9.11 The Cat stretch

Chopping   This following movement will exercise the sacral area and the muscles exerted in childbirth. It also affects the milk glands and so will be good to do even after delivery.

- Squat down with your feet flat on the floor. Clasp your hands together and make a chopping movement up over the head with your arms, which should be kept straight. Look at your hands as you bring them up over your head (*see* fig. 9.12). Follow up with the next exercise, the Pump.

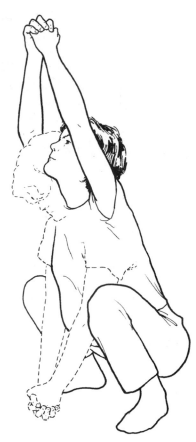

fig. 9.12 Chopping

The Pump • Stay in the squatting position and place your arms on the inside of your legs with your finger in under your insteps. Breathe in and, on the exhalation, stretch your legs as much as you can, letting your head drop down.

• Inhale again and return to squatting position, looking upwards. Repeat five to ten times (*see* fig. 9.13). The Pump will help relax your back and release blocked energy in your pelvic region.

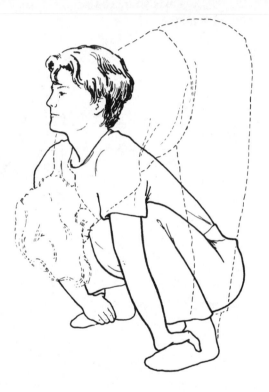

fig. 9.13 The Pump

Lie down on your back on the floor for the next two exercises, which will work on strengthening your abdominal muscles and aligning your pelvis:

• Keep your knees bent and open to the sides. Bend your arms and bring your elbows to the floor on the side of your body with your fists clenched. Take a deep breath in and, as you breathe out, press your elbows against the floor and raise your chest up towards the ceiling, still with your knees apart (*see* fig. 9.14). Come back to the starting position as you inhale. Repeat three or four times.

- Lie on your back with your legs in the same position as above. Bring your hands together in front of your chest, with your fingers pointed up towards your chin and your forearms parallel to the floor. Take a deep breath in and, as you exhale, straighten your arms up above your head at the same time as you stretch your legs out. Try to keep your hands and feet together (*see* fig. 9.15). Come back to your starting position on the next inhalation and repeat the exercise another three or four times.

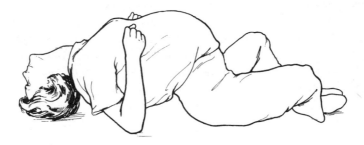

fig. 9.14 Strengthening exercise for abdominal muscles

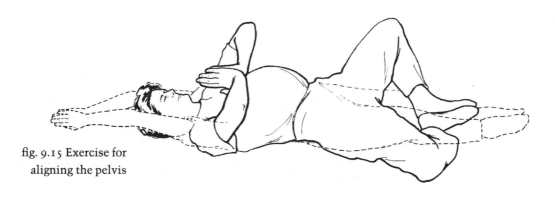

fig. 9.15 Exercise for aligning the pelvis

Lie down on your back with your arms at the side and allow yourself to relax immediately after performing this set of exercises.

Miscarriage

Traditionally in Japan a pregnant woman would use the contraindicated points discussed earlier to assure herself that the pregnancy was healthy. If this was not the case, the foetus would naturally abort after the stimulation of these points. Today we strongly recommend not using these points, as it may cause a miscarriage.

In Oriental medicine, we distinguish between six different types of miscarriage, with various symptoms, all requiring different treatments to help prevent a miscarriage and also better prepare a woman for future pregnancies after a miscarriage:

- General Ki Deficiency – *frequent vaginal bleeding, fainting, abdominal swelling, aversion to cold and a poor appetite. General tonification through shiatsu is needed here.*
- Blood Deficiency – *the dropping of the lower hara, swelling, dizziness, a yellow complexion, puffiness, a weak pulse and palpitations. Get your partner to treat your Spleen, Kidney, Heart and Liver meridians (as described in Chapter 5), to tone the Blood.*
- Kidney Deficiency – *vaginal bleeding, back pain (lumbar), water retention and frequent urination. Tonify the Kidney and Spleen meridians.*
- Hot Blood – *menstrual-type flow, a bright red or red complexion, heat in the upper body, cold feet, a sore and dry throat and scanty, hot urine. Treat the Kidney, Lung and Spleen meridians.*
- Liver Ki congestion – *painful foetal motion, vaginal bleeding, vomiting or a bilious taste, a thick and greasy yellow coating on the tongue and a rapid pulse. Treat the Liver meridian and release the diaphragm as described on pages 154–5; tonify the Kidney and Spleen meridians.*
- Traumatic injury – *this is an external causation and you should seek professional attention.*

To prepare yourself for future pregnancy, a change in diet is sometimes necessary (*see* advice on diet on page 153 under Second Trimester and on pages 138–40 under Are You Underweight or Overweight?) Support the energy flow in the meridian system by practising general Do-In and meridian stretching exercises (*see* Chapter 7), and tone up your pelvic area by doing the pelvic floor exercises (*see* page 147).

Childbirth and Pain Relief

Childbirth is the culmination of your pregnancy – the moment to which all your preparations during the last nine months have been leading. Knowing about the different stages of labour will, to a certain extent, help to control any fear and discomfort. As you gain information and understanding about the birth process, your self-confidence will increase and you will be able to use the different exercises and breathing techniques to release some of the pain and, hopefully, enjoy giving birth.

Even if every birth is unique and has its own individual timetable, labour can be divided into three well-defined stages. We will now give a brief explanation of the course of events and describe how shiatsu can help you through the different stages.

The First Stage of Labour

The first stage of labour can last from several hours to a day or more. During this first stage the cervix opens out (or dilates) fully, to allow space for your baby's head to pass through. The period usually starts with a show of mucus or the rupture of the water membranes. Your contractions will gradually become longer and stronger, with shorter intervals between each one. In this phase of labour your Yang is going into Excess, expressed as greater body heat and activity. You are fully dilated when your cervix has opened to ten centimetres (four inches), and you then move gradually into the second stage of labour.

During this first stage what is most important is to relax. When you relax you support the Yang by strengthening the Yin: breathe slowly and allow your body to do its work. This is usually quite easy for the first part and a lot of women choose to walk around and be active between contractions. When the cervix is about half-dilated, it might get harder. You will benefit now from resting and regaining some energy between your contractions. Choose a position comfortable for you – perhaps a side position with the knees slightly bent. This position enables your partner to apply pressure to the sacral area, using the thumbs or the palm of their hand. Move into the indentations of the sacrum, applying firm pressure and rotating the thumb at the same time.

Speeding a Slow Labour
If the labour is slow, you can use the following tsubo to speed it up: SP 6, LIV 3, BL 31, LI 4 and GB 21 (see fig. 9.16). General Do-In and the different squatting exercises described earlier will also be beneficial.

173

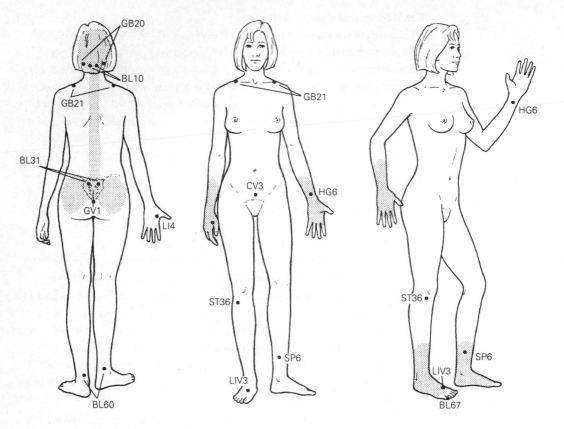

fig. 9.16 Labour: point
location chart

Feeling Like Giving Up?	If your energy is decreasing and you feel like giving up, Ginseng or *Ume-sho-bancha* tea (*see* page 156) will help you regain some strength. Get your partner to treat your Kidney meridian and apply pressure to ST 36 below your knee (*see* fig. 9.16).
When Labour Is Overdue or 'Lazy'	Generally speaking, unless there is foetal distress, the pregnancy should be allowed to continue without intervention. Each day of growth strengthens your child. If there is a 'need' to stimulate labour, try the following:

Stimulate LI 4, SP 6, GB 21 and BL 67 (*see* fig. 9.16). If there is no response in six to eight hours, try stimulating the above points again, adding GV 1. Hot, spicy food has an expelling affect, as it is very Yang in quality, so eat an Indian takeaway and perform some general Do-In exercises.

174

Shiatsu for Pregnancy and Childbirth

The Second Stage of Labour
The second stage of labour usually lasts for one to three hours and ends with the birth of your baby. You now start to play a more active role in your labour and you will experience an instinctive feeling of wanting to push down. This is the stage where the baby is pushed through the cervix and vagina, leaving the womb to be born into this world.

Relieving Backache   This stage is less painful but does involve strenuous work. Stay in a side position to give your partner the opportunity to alleviate some of the pain in your back by rubbing the lower back and applying pressure to sacral and lumbar points.

Pain Relief   The pain of your contractions may become unbearable and beyond your 'control' and it will be very tempting to take advantage of the painkillers on offer. There are, however, certain tsubo which will help you regain your control of the pain. These may also have the effect of relaxing and shortening the contractions, so they should only be used when the pain is extreme. To use them too frequently may extend the labour. ST 36 and BL 60 are pain-relieving points; pressing into the sacrum will also assist in pain control (*see* fig. 9.16).

A semi-upright or squatting position will give you the force of gravity to help expel your baby. The contractions are involuntary and you will help the uterus by pushing during the contractions. Try to relax your pelvic floor muscles and to breathe deeply between the contractions. A gentle neck squeeze between contractions can be nice to relieve some of the neck tension. It will also ease the pelvis. GB 20 and BL 10 are good points to use.

The Third Stage of Labour
After your baby is born, the uterus takes a short 'rest' and then starts to contract again to expel the placenta. The placenta separates from the wall of the womb and comes out with the amniotic sac. This is usually a painless process and you can enjoy the opportunity of attending to your baby in the meantime. Seeing, touching and putting your baby to the breast will help in the production of oxytocin (a hormone that increases the contractions of the uterus and speeds up the process of expelling the placenta).

Releasing the Placenta   If there is a problem with retention of the placenta, get your partner to apply pressure to HG 6, GB 21, CV 3, BL 60, LI 4 and SP 6. You could also try blowing into an empty bottle (*see* fig. 9.16).

Help after Childbirth
Take a Break – You Deserve It!
Allow yourself a few days of complete rest from anything other than attending to your newborn baby. Take the opportunity to rest and sleep when your baby is sleeping. You will need time to recover from the hard work of childbirth and these first days are really important for bonding with your baby. A full shiatsu treatment from your partner will ease any muscular soreness and help restore energy.

You will continue to feel quite strong contractions from the uterus for a few days after the birth. This is a good sign and shows that your uterus is getting back to its normal size again. You will also experience a discharge of mucus and blood from the uterus (lochia), which will go on for anything up to six weeks. Use sanitary pads rather than tampons for the first couple of weeks after the delivery.

Both processes above will be shorter if you breast-feed your baby. Breast-feeding stimulates the production of the hormones that causes the uterus and other structures (such as the ligaments that control your pelvic girdle and hip socket) to shrink. This process is initiated by the strong sucking stimulation to ST 17 (the nipple) and the meridian connected to the ovaries.

Improving Lactation
Breast-feeding is important for the bonding between mother and child. It will help build up your baby's immune system, reduce the risk of allergies and support the growth and development of your child. Successful breast-feeding is dependent on your ability to produce a steady flow of milk. Shiatsu treatments will ease any tension and worries you might have and help relax the breast muscles.

Treatment   There are particular tsubo you can stimulate to improve poor lactation. Use the following tsubo in combination with a general soothing massage of your breasts: SP18, LIV 14, ST 13, 16 and 17, HG 1, SI 11 and CV 17 (*see* fig. 9.17).

The 'release' of milk is stimulated by the hormone oxytocin, which in turn is stimulated by breast-feeding. Encouraging your baby to suck will, therefore, increase the amount of milk you produce. Allow yourself enough time when feeding, as stress of any kind will negatively affect the production of milk. Avoid caffeine and drink herbal tea instead – spearmint or peppermint, for example.

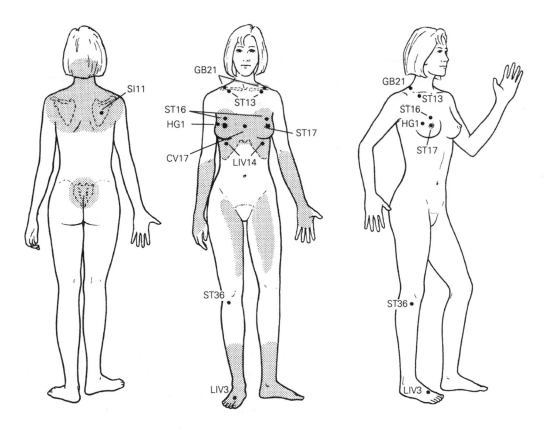

fig. 9.17 Improving lactation/mastitis: point location chart

Mastitis
This occurs when infection enters the breast, usually through a cracked nipple. Your breast will become hard, red and tender. To avoid cracking, apply some *Calendula* or Vitamin E oil to your nipples and allow them to dry properly before putting your bra on after you have fed your baby.

Treatment   In Oriental terms, this is classified as a 'hot disease' and an Excess condition. To help bring energy down in the body, massage your breasts and armpits. Use the following tsubo: ST 18 and 36, GB 21, LIV 3 and 14, SI 11 and CV 17 (*see* fig. 9.17). Warm your lower abdomen with a hot water bottle.

Perineal Pain or Post-Episiotomy

Episiotomy (an incision made in the perineum between the vaginal opening and the anus) is a common operation in the Western world, performed to allow the pelvic floor muscles to relax and the perineum to bulge to avoid a tear. A good semi-upright position during the second stage of labour will help to avoid the need for an episiotomy, which unfortunately can lead to bruising, swelling and a great deal of pain and discomfort. If you do tear or decide to have an episiotomy, here are some suggestions for treatment afterwards.

Treatment   Apply an ice pack to your perineum directly after the birth of your baby (for 5–10 minutes). Follow up with alternatively bathing it in hot and cold water. Sea-salt baths (place a handful of sea salt in your bath water) are very good, and you can also apply some *Calendula* or wheat-germ oil if the area feels dry and itchy. To help bruising, take the homoeopathic remedy *Arnica*.

Postnatal Depression

This may be a physical or emotional response to giving birth. Hormonal changes occurring after childbirth can sometimes upset the psychological and emotional state of the mother. This ranges from mild depression to extreme feelings of isolation and anxiety. Receiving shiatsu from your partner or a professional therapist is the best approach, combined with openly expressing your feelings, whether these be anger, pain, fear or disappointment. 'Can I be a good mother?' is not an easy question to answer and requires encouragement and support from your partner or friends.

Treatment   There is no easy self-treatment equation other than to try to rest and nurture yourself and your baby as well as possible. Complete rest for at least one month will speed your recovery and ensure the better production of breast milk. It will help improve your strength to care for your child. Try to get help from friends and relatives to enable you to take this rest. Practise your full-body Do-In exercises each day, together with the body scrubs described in Chapter 7.

Strengthening Exercises
You should start to do some gentle exercises as soon as possible after the birth of your child. You will be able to practise the first few exercises described here while lying in bed.

Exercises to Strengthen your Stomach Muscles

1) Lie on your back with your knees bent and your hands resting on your abdomen. Take a deep breath in and, as you exhale, press your back into the bed. You will feel your abdominal muscles tightening up underneath your hands. Hold for a while, then relax. Repeat ten times.

2) Do the pelvic floor exercise as described in Chapter 8. This will help tune up the internal organs, bring energy into the pelvic region and help stimulate circulation in the area.

3) Lying on your back, bring your knees up to your chest and gently press them down. Breathe in deeply and, on the exhalation, bring your forehead to your knees. Hold for 10–15 seconds and then relax down again. This will strengthen your abdominal muscles and stretch your back. Repeat five to ten times (*see* fig. 9.18).

4) When you feel up to it, start doing the following curl ups: lie on your back with your knees bent and your hands resting on your thighs. Breathe in and, on the exhalation, raise your head and shoulders and reach for your knees with your hands. Hold the position for 10–15 seconds and then relax. Repeat as many times as you can.

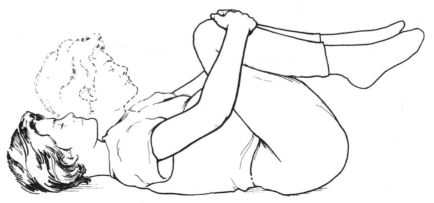

fig. 9.18
Abdominal muscles strengthening exercise

179

Exercises for Pelvic and Spinal Alignment

1) Crawling on all fours is one of the best exercises for your back. Practise a bit of crawling and then do the Cat Stretch exercise described on page 168.

2) Lying on your back, relax your right arm out to the side of your body. Bend your right leg and put the foot onto your left knee. Breathe in and, on the exhalation, slowly bring the right knee over to the left side, using your left hand as support on top of the left knee (*see* fig. 9.19). Turn your head to the right and try to keep the right shoulder on the floor. Inhale and return to starting position. Repeat with the left leg and then repeat twice on both sides.

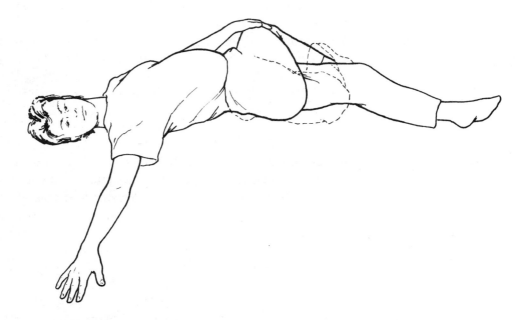

fig. 9.19 Exercise for pelvic and spinal alignment

Keep practising the above exercises for a couple of weeks after the delivery. As you begin to feel stronger, start your Do-In exercises and try to build up a regular daily exercise routine. It is more beneficial to do a little every day than to save it all for one day a week.

chapter 10

Self-Treatments for Gynaecological Problems

We have listed here a number of common problems which may be assisted by shiatsu self-treatment. Please refer to the details of how to apply pressure and the information about determining if a tsubo or area is in a Kyo or Jitsu condition (*see* Chapter 3). You will then be in a position to decide whether to tonify the Kyo tsubo with patient holding pressure of about 10–15 seconds, or to sedate a Jitsu tsubo with a stronger, stimulating, movement-type treatment. Check each tsubo listed for how it feels and experiment; does it feel better to 'hold it' or is it more satisfying to 'move it'? Trust your own intuition.

It is always best to treat the whole meridian wherever possible and to receive a full-body treatment regularly to ensure the best results. Where we have indicated a series of tsubo to treat, it is best to treat these in the order that they appear. You may find that some tsubo 'feel right', while others don't give you any immediate response. Concentrate on the former.

The Menstrual Cycle Energetics
The Chinese historically considered the menstrual cycle or 'Moon Flow' to be a natural reflection of the natural order of change. Everything is in continual movement, changing from Excess to Deficiency, Yang to Yin. As we have already mentioned, the Chinese refer to the womb as a 'Blood

Chamber' where menstrual blood is produced to enhance the womb environment ready for conception, should you choose to have a child. The production and elimination of the menstrual blood also help to maintain blood quality control for your whole body. As the blood builds up, it reaches an Excess and, if conception has not occurred, the blood will discharge as your 'Heavenly Water' when the Blood Chamber goes into Deficiency. This is why your energy levels fluctuate at this time. The whole process then starts again (*see* fig. 10.1).

fig. 10.1 The cycle of menstruation with phases of Excess and Deficiency

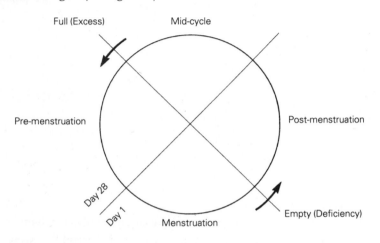

When all is in order there is no pain, so pain or other discomforts indicate an imbalance. Remember, any discomfort relating to the reproductive system is a reflection of your whole being, so try not to think of your reproductive organs as a separate entity which you dislike during menstruation. Try to see your reproductive system as a part of the whole and think about the wonders of your body and what potential you can achieve.

Please note for reference to all illustrations:
All tsubo are bilaterally located on the body unless found on the midline. Shaded areas indicate where to give general shiatsu treatment.

Abdominal Bloating

Abdominal bloating is due to the excess fluid accumulating in the peritoneal cavity of your abdomen and, most commonly, occurs just before menstruation. It is a stagnant Blood and Ki condition and shows a Deficiency in the Lower Burner. It therefore involves Liver Ki stagnation. Oedema may also cause abdominal bloating (*see* pages 162 and 203).

Treatment
Follow the advice under Oedema and gently massage your lower abdomen, paying special attention to the cv channel. Apply pressure to the following points: LIV 3 and 6, SP 12 and 15, ST 36, KID 1 and 27, BL 16, 17 and 25 (*see* fig. 10.2).

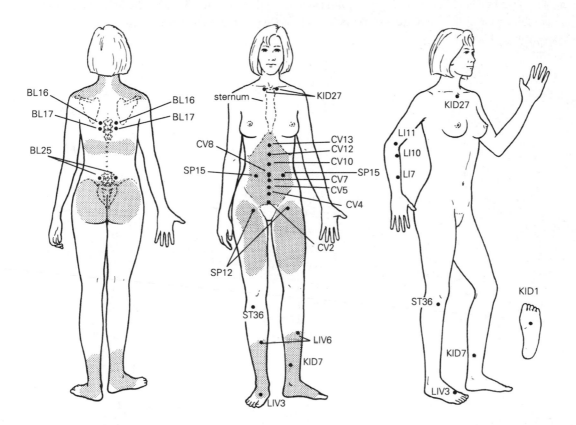

fig. 10.2 Abdominal bloating: point location chart

Amenorrhoea

This is the stoppage or absence of menstruation. Another symptom can be very slight periods. Here we differentiate between primary and secondary amenorrhoea.

Primary amenorrhoea is defined as a failure to start menstruating by the age of 16. The main reason for this is the delayed onset of puberty, which in itself can be due to eating disorders such as bulimia, anorexia nervosa, excessive eating or starvation, any or all of which may affect your hormonal production and balance. If you do not feed yourself properly, your Spleen energy will be depleted and the Spleen is one of the organ functions involved with the production of Blood. Clearly, to be able to menstruate, you need to produce an Excess of Blood.

Everything you eat and drink is first received by the Stomach, which in Chinese Medicine is likened to a pot on a stove. As the food is 'cooked'

fig. 10.3 Amenorrhoea: point location chart

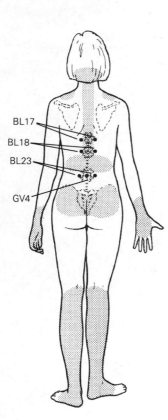
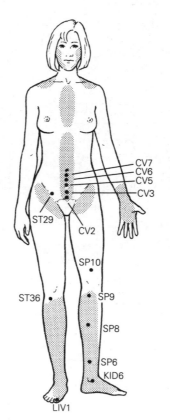
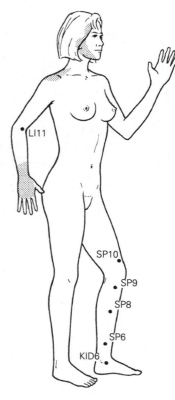

by the Stomach, it is 'rottened and ripened'. This Stomach activity prepares the ground for the Spleen to separate and extract a refined Essence from food and drink. This is called the Grain (Nutritive) Ki and is the basis for the production of Ki and Blood. The Spleen takes this refined Essence and 'sends' it up to the Heart, where it mixes with the Essence from the Kidneys and is transformed into Blood. The Heart then pumps out the Blood to the rest of the body. As mentioned before, menstrual Blood is Excess Blood sent down to the uterus. The uterus is closely connected to the Liver which 'stores' the Blood. If the Liver properly stores adequate Blood, menstruation occurs on schedule and is normal in volume.

Other possible causes for primary amenorrhoea are emotional stress and too much rigorous exercise. This will also affect your Spleen energy in a negative way. If a girl has not begun her periods by 16 or 17 years of age, it is possible (but rare) that she may have congenital abnormalities of the genital organs or endocrine system function and so should seek further medical investigation into this.

Secondary amenorrhoea is the temporary or permanent cessation of periods in a woman who has menstruated regularly in the past. This is a normal consequence of pregnancy or breast-feeding. Periods may also cease temporarily after a woman has stopped taking oral contraceptives; they usually return after six to eight weeks but may not do so for a year or longer in some cases. Secondary amenorrhoea can also result from hormonal changes due to emotional stress, depression, eating disorders such as those mentioned above, or certain drugs. Strenuous exercise, such as long-distance running, may also influence your periods in a negative way.

Treatment

Nourish yourself through a well-balanced diet. Foods that are naturally sweet and/or pungent – well-cooked rice, sweet rice, oats and millet, for example – are excellent ('sweet' does not include table sugar). Other beneficial foods include: carbohydrate-rich vegetables such as winter squash, carrots, parsnips, sweet potatoes, yam, pumpkins and turnips; pungent vegetables and spices such as onions, leeks, ginger, cinnamon, garlic, fennel and nutmeg. All food should be cooked (but not overcooked) and chewed well, as chewing physically breaks down the food and, through chewing, you stimulate the production of saliva which starts the chemical breakdown of the food.

Stimulate your Spleen meridian in the leg and focus on the following tsubo: SP 6, 8, 9 and 10 (*see* fig. 10.3). The tsubo below your navel on the CV channel will also prove very beneficial for treating amenorrhoea, so apply pressure to the individual tsubo (CV 2, 3, 5, 6 and 7) or just gently massage

Shiatsu for Women

down the centre line below your navel. CV 1, located at the centre of your perineum (between the anus and vagina), can be stimulated by using your heel as you sit down on the floor in a crossed-leg position. Stimulate the Reproductive Point in the buttock area using tennis balls (*see* Chapter 3) or your fists. Other beneficial tsubo include: KID 6 and ST 36, BL 17, 18 and 23, LI 11 and GV 4 (*see* fig. 10.3).

Breast Lumps
Breast lumps are what we commonly call any mass, cyst or swelling that can be felt in the breast tissue. It is very important that you self-examine your breasts every month, to feel for any changes in your breasts and check if there is any discharge from your nipples. If you find any lumps or discharge, contact your doctor immediately.

There are many different types of breast lumps; about 80 per cent of them are of benign character (not cancerous) and the rest are malignant.

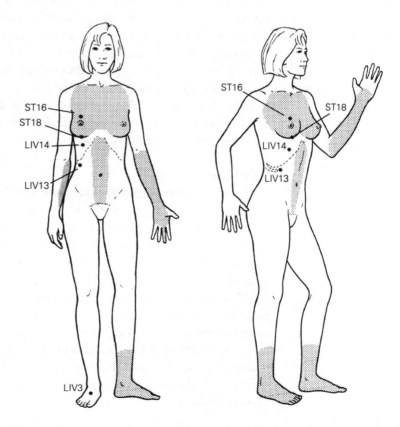

fig. 10.4 Breast lumps: point location chart

186

Your doctor might suggest a mammography or have a biopsy taken to find out what kind of growth you have. Once you know what is there, you can make a decision as to what to do and how to treat it.

Treatment
As a lump or swelling is usually a sign of stagnation, we recommend that you treat your Liver meridian in the legs, focusing on LIV 3, 13 and 14. Gently massage your breasts and nipples and treat the points on the Stomach meridian: ST 16 and 18. For improving circulation, treat your Heart and Heart Governor meridians in the arms (*see* fig. 10.4).

Lumps that are softer, tender, not painful to touch, come and go with your menstruation and are better after massage are due to Liver Ki stagnation. Lumps that are more fixed, painful to touch, do not respond to massage or your menstrual cycle are caused by Blood stasis – an obstruction of Blood. This latter condition requires professional medical advice.

Cystitis

Most women suffer from cystitis at some point in their lives. It is usually caused by a bacterial infection. Since the urethra is short, it is easy for different infectious agents to pass from the vagina or anus up into the bladder.

External Pernicious Influences such as Cold and Damp may also cause cystitis. Cold from the outside penetrates the internal environment and the body's reaction to this is to activate your internal Fire. You might experience symptoms such as frequent, painful or burning urinations. The burning sensation tells you that there is Heat in the system and a good precaution against this is to avoid Cold getting into the area – so do not sit on cold surfaces or allow the area to get cold and wet. Do you remember your mother telling you to get out of your swimming costume after a swim? Now you know why. Wear warm, natural-fibre underwear in the winter (synthetics disturb your Ki flow), to help prevent cystitis.

Treatment
If you are suffering from cystitis, try to warm your lower abdomen by using a hot-water bottle on the area below the navel. Sea-salt baths will also be very good and, if the burning and itching is bad, use some natural yoghurt externally and internally to cool the area down. This is Yin putting out the Yang Fire. Apply pressure to the following tsubo: ST 36, BL 20, 23, 25 and 27, CV 3, 4 and 5 (*see* fig. 10.5 overleaf).

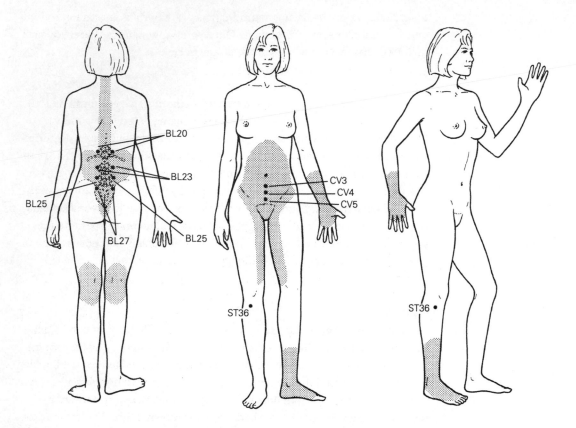

fig. 10.5 Cystitis: point
location chart

Dysmenorrhoea

If dysmenorrhoea or menstrual cramping commenced in your teenage
years with your early periods, it is referred to as *Primary dysmenorrhoea*.
At this tender age, your reproductive hormones were excitedly blossoming
ready for womanhood and your stress levels would have had a direct effect
on hormonal production.

Prostaglandins or 'local hormones' will most likely affect your menstrual cramping. These hormones cause muscular contractions of the
uterus and, when overstimulated, they can spread throughout the pelvic
organs wantonly causing contractions in many areas. So why does this
happen? Mostly as a result of stress or there may have been some physical
or emotional shock or trauma which upset your energy system either early
in childhood or as an adult. Even birth trauma, such as a protracted labour
or a careless forceps delivery, could create undue internal pressures in the
cranium, hence stressing your endocrine system.

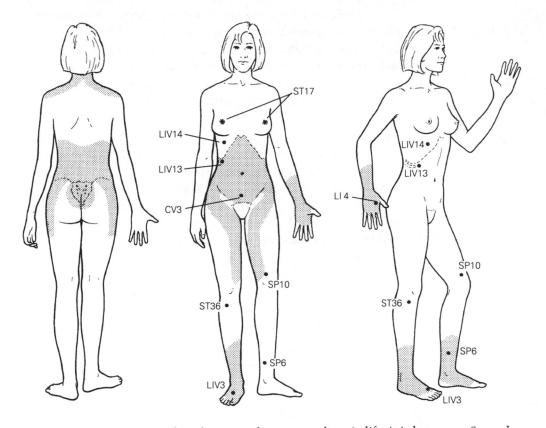

fig. 10.6 Dysmenorrhoea: point location chart

When dysmenorrhoea occurs later in life, it is known as *Secondary dysmenorrhoea* and different factors require consideration. Stress of course does not only occur in adolescence and it may well affect you throughout your adult life. You may have been influenced by the use of the contraceptive pill or interuterine device (IUD), both of which can have detrimental effects. Your hormonal system is influenced by the Kidney Ki and is especially sensitive to fear and anxiety which disturb the free flow of the Ki. The uterus and its environment is regulated by the Liver and Spleen Ki. The Liver Ki is responsible for Blood storage and regulation as well as the muscular contraction impetus, and the Spleen Ki for the quality of the 'flesh' of the uterus. Other factors influencing the Moon Cycle would be the invasion of Cold and Damp into your body. This may be an accumulative effect of foods such as sugars, caffeine or dairy products, which all cause Ki stagnation.

Of course you may have an External Pernicious Influence to combat. Living in a cold, damp, basement flat will injure your protective energy

189

(Wei Ki) and immune system. If you don't take preventative measures, it will just keep spreading. Always keep your pelvis well-insulated with natural-fibre clothing during colder periods. The ankles (which swell in some women during or preceding menstruation) have a special relationship to your reproductive system, so it is important to keep them warm as well. Warm socks and warm shoes will help here.

Treatment

Apply pressure to the following tsubo: LIV 3, SP 6 and 10, and ST 36 (*see* fig. 10.6) You may even strap a stainless steel ball bearing or a grain of uncooked rice to SP 6 (*see* fig. 10.6) for one or two days at the time of usual cramping. Also apply pressure to the following tsubo: CV 3, LIV 13 and 14, and LI 4 (*see* fig. 10.6). Massage your nipples as this will stimulate the ovaries and, using your fingertips, gently massage the area between your pubic bone and the navel.

Using the tennis balls as described in Chapter 3, roll them along your lumbar spine and generally under the buttocks and sacrum, for BL 32 especially (*see* fig. 10.7). If you want firmer pressure, use golf balls under the sacrum and buttocks instead. Do pelvic floor exercise as described in

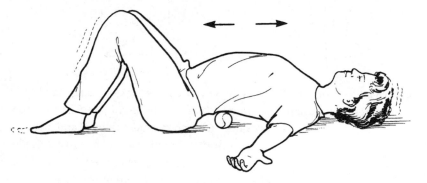

fig. 10.7 Self-treatment of sacrum and buttocks

Chapter 8. Heat (Yang) is relaxing for the cramping contraction (Yin), so a hot-water bottle on your abdomen helps to expel the symptoms of the Cold and Damp. Apply the meridian stretches and other exercises for the Spleen, Liver and Kidney shown in Chapter 7. Avoid stimulants such as coffee, cigarettes, sugar and chemicalized foods, to allow your energy system to repair.

Endometriosis

This is a condition where fragments of the inner lining of the uterus (the endometrium) grow in abnormal places outside of it, most commonly in the Fallopian tubes, the ovaries or behind the uterus. These misplaced parts of the endometrium will continue to respond to the menstrual cycle and hormonal changes as if they were still inside the uterus. Common symptoms include painful and heavy menstruation, lower back and abdominal pain, and pain during sexual intercourse. In some cases, endometriosis will be asymptomatic – that is, there are no symptoms at all. Why or how endometriosis causes infertility is still unknown to Western medicine and 30–40 per cent of infertile women suffer from this condition.

Pain during intercourse is an important symptom confirming Blood stagnation – endometriosis is a Blood stagnation condition. There are four basic patterns to look at[1]: Ki congestion and Blood stagnation; Blood stagnation due to accumulation of Cold; Heat congestion with Blood stagnation; and Blood and Ki Deficiency with Blood stagnation. As this is such a complex condition, it is recommended to seek professional help for a

fig. 10.8 Endometriosis: point location chart

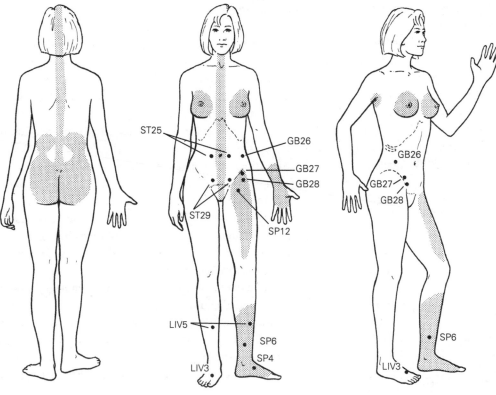

course of shiatsu treatments. However, here are a few suggestions on what you can do for yourself between sessions with your practitioner.

Treatment
Stimulate the Liver and Spleen meridians in your legs and treat the following tsubo: LIV 3 and 5, GB 26, 27 and 28, SP 4, 6 and 12, ST 25 and 29 (*see* fig. 10.8). Use a tennis ball to stimulate the Reproductive Point in your buttocks and body scrub daily to stimulate the circulation and movement of Blood. Use the visualization techniques described in Chapter 7 to release the stagnation and also try some affirmations.

Fibroids

These are benign tumours of the muscle wall of the uterus. The word 'fibroid' is rather misleading, as the tumour cells are not in fact fibrous but instead consist of abnormal, smooth muscle bundles and connective tissue which grow slowly within the uterine wall. As a fibroid enlarges, it may grow within the muscle, so that the uterine cavity is distorted. Fibroids may be as small as a pea or as large as a grapefruit, and there may be one or more of them. They are among the most common tumours, occurring in about 20 per cent of women over 30. The cause of fibroids is unknown in Western medicine, although some studies indicate that they might be hereditary. It is also thought that fibroids are related to an abnormal response to oestrogen hormones[2], so oral contraceptives containing oestrogen may cause fibroids to enlarge, as can pregnancy.

Very often fibroids are asymptomatic, especially if the fibroid is small. This makes fibroids difficult to diagnose yourself and you might need an ultrasound scanning to confirm the diagnosis. The most common symptoms include heavy periods and bleeding between periods, painful menstruation, painful sexual intercourse and/or bleeding after intercourse. There might be swelling of the lower abdomen and quite often lower back pain. As you are loosing more blood than normal, you might become anaemic and feel tired and pale. Fibroids that distort the uterine cavity may be responsible for recurrent miscarriage and infertility.

This is a condition where the Blood and Ki has stagnated and so you want to relieve this stagnation. 'When Ki moves, Blood follows', 'If Ki stagnates, Blood congeals' are Oriental sayings which show the relationship between Blood and Ki. If Ki is stagnant, it will not be able to move the Blood as 'Ki is the commander of Blood'. According to Oriental Medicine, this can be due to long-standing emotional problems, such as resentment, anger and frustration.

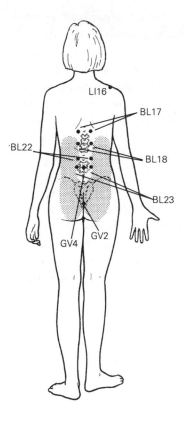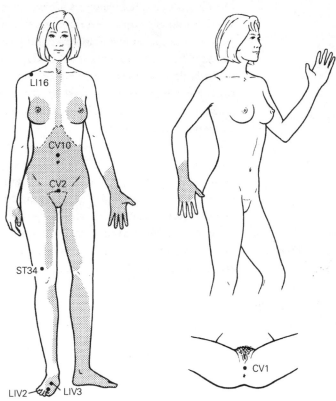

fig. 10.9 Fibroids: point
location chart

Treatment
Use the following tsubo to remove the stasis: CV 1, 2 and 10, GV 2 and 4,
LIV 2 and 3, BL 17, 18, 22, 23 and 31–4 (in the sacrum), ST 34 and LI 16
(*see* fig. 10.9).

Infertility

In Oriental Medicine, female infertility is called *Bu Yun Zheng*, which
means 'no pregnancy condition'. As already mentioned, traditionally infertility was treated with the belief that conception takes place as a result of
mixing the woman's 'red essence' (vaginal blood) with the 'white essence'
(sperm) from the man. Anything that might lead to Deficient Blood or stagnation of Blood can therefore cause infertility. There might be many different reasons for this to happen, both on a physical, emotional or
psychological level.

193

According to Bob Flaws,[3] there are 12 different causes to look for, from the Chinese viewpoint, the three most common of which are a misplaced womb, obesity and being underweight (*see* Chapter 7). However, infertility can also be due to abdominal obstruction, the emotions of jealousy, anger and self-pity, or poor circulation. As this is such a complex condition, it is recommended to go for a course of treatments with a professional shiatsu practitioner. However, here are some suggestions for how to treat yourself between your treatments.

Treatment
Make sure you give yourself time for regular exercise and relaxation throughout your week. Eat a well-balanced diet and body scrub every day (see Chapter 7). Get your partner to give you full-body shiatsu for relaxation every now and then, and bring special attention to the following tsubo: CV 3 and GV 4 (the area on the back in level with the navel is considered a corridor for the Source Ki, Kidney Ki and Essence), GV 20, SP 6 and 8,

fig. 10.10 Infertility: point location chart

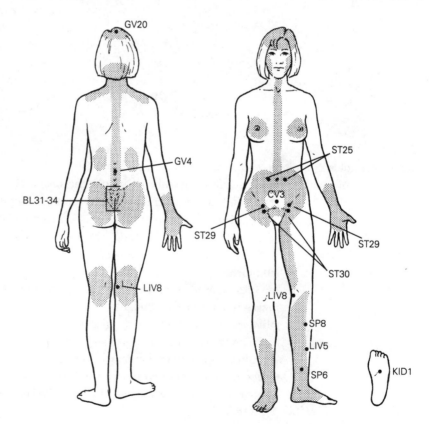

194

LIV 5 and 8, ST 25 and 29 (the name of this point is *Return*, which refers to its influence on the menstrual cycle and its ability to restore the tissue and position of the uterus to normal) and ST 30, BL 31–4 and KID 1 (the name *Gushing Spring*, suggests this point's fresh and active energy) (*see* fig. 10.10).

Menopausal Disturbances

Menopause usually occurs between the ages of 45–55. Due to a reduced production of oestrogen, the monthly menstruation stops and you will notice changes both physically and psychologically. When you have missed 12 consecutive periods, the menopausal process is completed. Before that you might experience scanty and irregular bleeding for a period of time.

Physical symptoms of the menopause might include: hot flushes and night sweats; vaginal dryness causing sexual intercourse to be more difficult and painful; and frequent urinations (a sign of a Yin Deficiency). On the psychological and emotional side, you might suffer from a lack of concentration, tearfulness and anxiety. Internal changes in your metabolism may also lead to osteoporosis (brittle bones) developing at a later stage.

It is very popular today to treat different menopausal discomforts with hormone replacement therapy (HRT). Unfortunately, HRT has had a lot of reported side effects and symptoms sometimes recur after treatment has been discontinued. No one really understands the best way to take this drug and there is little control over the amount of oestrogen released into the bloodstream.[4] To take it orally sometimes gives side effects such as nausea, vomiting, cramps or bloating, and the skin patch might lead to blistering and discoloration of the skin. Using oestrogen alone increases the risk of endometrial cancer up to 20-fold. Therefore, many women are given progestogen to counteract the oestrogen. Unfortunately, this can also cause side effects such as tender breasts, cramps, bloating, depression, anxiety and irritability – symptoms which HRT was supposed to treat in the first place. Progestogen may also increase the risk of breast cancer. These are just some of the side effects women might suffer from taking HRT, which will eventually create an Internal Cold condition leading to Blood stagnation.

The many different menopausal 'distress' symptoms can all be treated and alleviated through shiatsu. Menopause is a natural process and it is never too late to start to focus on self-care, in combination with some appropriate treatments. Keep up your daily exercise programme and follow the suggestions overleaf.

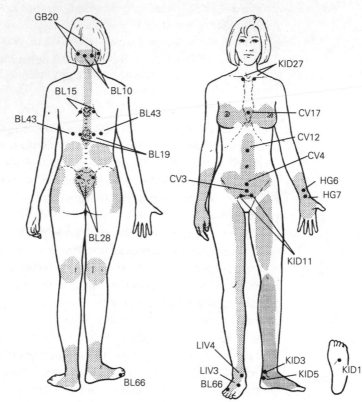

fig. 10.11 Menopause:
point location chart

Treatment
- *Hot flushes and night sweats*: BL 10, 28 and 43, GB 20, CV 3, 4, 12 and 17, KID 3 and 5 (*see* fig. 10.11).
- *Vaginal changes and dryness*: reduce your intake of sugar and practise the pelvic floor exercises in Chapter 8. Apply wheat-germ oil to the inside of your vagina and use the following tsubo: KID 1, 3 and 11, and BL 66 (*see* fig. 10.11).
- *Anxiety:* treat your Heart Governor meridian on the inside of your arms and apply pressure to HG 6 and 7, KID 27 and BL 43 (*see* fig. 10.11).
- *Irritability*: treat your Liver and Gall Bladder meridian and practise different hip movement exercises (*see* Chapter 7) to release the stagnant energy in the pelvic area. Apply pressure to the following tsubo: LIV 3 and 4, and BL 15 (*see* fig. 10.11).

Menstrual Irregularity

A good question to ask yourself is, 'Is the rest of my life regular?' If your lifestyle is erratic and active in a stressful way, then do not be surprised if your body responds accordingly. A happy woman will have a happy menstrual cycle. So where has it all gone wrong? Time for reflection and change perhaps. Positive thoughts and a regulated lifestyle will help regulate your periods.

The relevant External Pernicious Influences may be loud, bright places with overwhelming smoky atmospheres and lots of frenetic people. Don't make this a regular hangout. Eat simply *most* of the time, try to get into a more regular sleep pattern to recharge your Kidney Ki (we wouldn't usually refer to two to ten in the morning as 'regular'), and introduce frequent exercise. Have fun without the need to dash about madly all over the place, pace yourself and just have the occasional spontaneous spurts of unadulterated pleasure rather than constant hormonal uprisings. Give yourself a few months and your cycle will return to normal.

The Spleen and Liver influences in particular are relevant here. The Spleen for its ability to 'hold' the blood and upwards-moving energies, as well as the psychological impression of your own self-image. The Liver for its 'storage' quality which, when overzealous, may create Heat and tension throughout the system.

There is no simple formula for deciding how to treat this problem since 'irregularity' has different causes and meanings. We will now look at these to help you decide which type you are.

A Short Cycle

A short cycle is usually an indication of Heat in your Blood and/or Ki depletion. The Heat syndrome is more Yang and so you may find heat in your lower abdomen; dark, clotting blood flow; dark urine; your tongue may be red with a yellow coating; and you may have a generally restless attitude caused by anxiety. Do you have a tendency to be hyperactive and then exhausted with heat rising to your head?

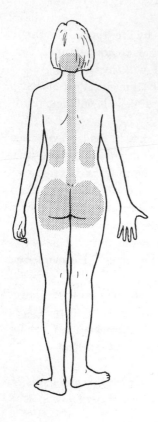
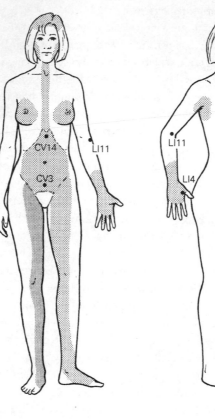

fig. 10.12 Short
menstrual cycle: point
location chart

Treatment   Cool the Blood and regulate the Kidney Ki as follows:
Apply pressure to the following tsubo: LI 4 and 11, CV 3 and 14 (*see* fig.
10.12). Reduce your alcohol consumption to a minimum to allow cooling
of the Liver Fire stress.

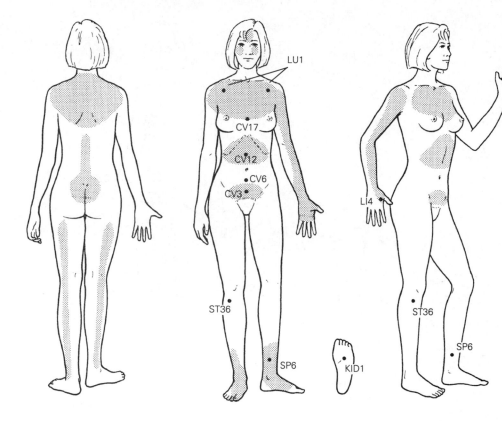

fig. 10.13 Ki depletion: point location chart

Ki Depletion

This will probably manifest itself as a profuse light and bright blood flow with a general emptiness in the lower abdomen, possibly bloating, general lethargy and breathlessness. Your tongue may be pale with a light, white coating.

Treatment Do general Do-In exercises and body scrubs with warm water daily (*see* Chapter 7) and apply pressure to the following tsubo: KID 1, SP 6, ST 36, LI 4, LU 1, and CV 3, 6, 12 and 17 (*see* fig. 10.12).

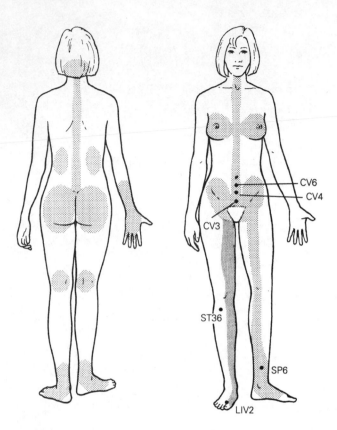

fig. 10.14 Late
menstruation: point
location chart

Late Menstruation

Late menstruation will express itself differently again and may be caused
by Blood depletion or a Coldness in the body, as well as a general sluggishness of the Ki flow (Ki stagnation). Blood depletion will probably manifest
itself with a scant and light red flow, a pale complexion, general lacklustre
skin with poor circulation, swelling or discomfort in the lower abdomen or
poor hair quality. Your tongue may be pink but have very little fur coating
and your pulse may feel weak.

Treatment   Regulate your eating patterns to include a good variety of foods,
especially white meat, fish two or three times weekly, and plenty of fresh
vegetables. Apply pressure to cv 4, 3 and 6, sp 6 and st 36 (*see* fig. 10.4). Do
deep-breathing exercises to improve blood oxygenation and nervous system
function (*see* Chapter 6), as well as the Do-In exercise routine daily. Pinch
the web between the big toe and second toe of each foot (liv 2), and generally
massage the area around your Achilles tendon (Kidney and Bladder points).

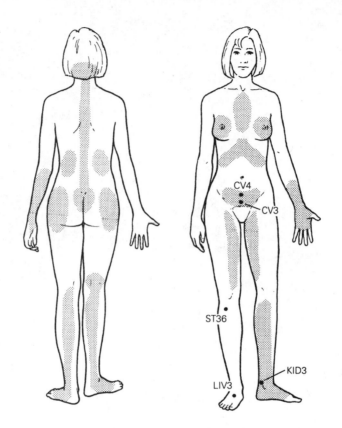

fig. 10.15 Cold Blood:
point location chart

Cold Blood

Cold Blood lacks the 'spark' of heat (Yang) necessary for harmonious blood flow. This may manifest itself as a dark, scanty blood flow, general coldness in the abdomen and buttocks, tightness and bloating in the lower abdomen, and cold extremities (you will probably find some relief in applying warmth to the abdomen). Your tongue may be pale with a thin, white fur coating, and the pulse will be quite slow and feel deep and difficult to locate.

Treatment Some general vigorous exercise would be good and also include the Do-In exercises from Chapter 7. Apply pressure to CV 3 and 4, ST 36, LIV 3 and KID 3 (*see* fig. 10.15).

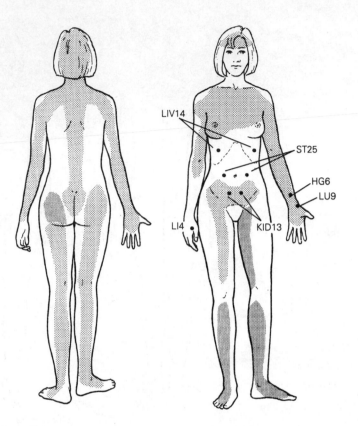

fig. 10.16 Ki stagnation:
point location chart

Ki Stagnation

This is a general condition requiring attention. When related to your menstrual cycle, however, it may manifest itself as the following: a scanty, dark blood flow with clotting; swollen ankles, abdomen and breasts; as well as general coldness in the extremities. There may also be some lethargy and depression and possible feelings of tightness in the chest or diaphragm, as the muscles are starved of oxygen and so restricted. Your tongue may be pale and have a thin, white coating and the pulse may feel rapid and tight, like a stretched wire.

Treatment Full-body exercises to improve your cardiovascular system and breathing potential will help stimulate the Ki, so take up regular walking, swimming, aerobics, jogging, cycling, gardening or active housework. Regulate your diet. Apply pressure to ST 25, KID 13, LIV 14, LU 9, HG 6 and LI 4 (*see* fig. 10.16).

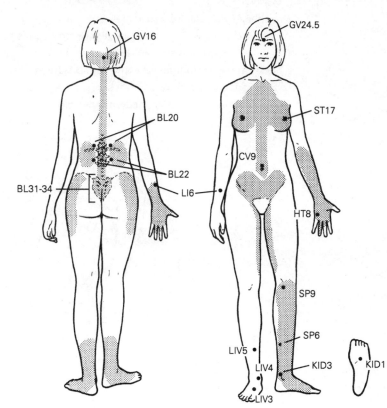

fig. 10.17 Oedema/
Ovarian cyst: point
location chart

Oedema

Oedema or water retention is a condition where fluid accumulates in and
around your cells, causing swelling in different parts of your body. Initially
oedema may show itself only as an increase in your weight. If the excess
fluid increases by more than 15 per cent, it then manifests itself as swelling,
most commonly in the lower part of the body (ankles, legs and the base of
the spine). Press a finger into the swollen area – the pressure will produce
an indentation in your skin, which slowly flattens out as the fluid returns.
This is classified as a Deficient Spleen symptom in Chinese Medicine. The
Spleen energy fails to transport fluids which therefore accumulate and in
turn obstruct the Kidney function of the transformation and excretion of
fluids. (*See also* page 162.)

Treatment
Add some natural diuretics to your diet, as these will stimulate water
loss and reduce the swelling in a natural way. Raw or steamed garlic and

cabbage will also be beneficial. Steep a teaspoon of dried parsley into a teacup of hot water and drink two or three cups per day.

CV 9 regulates the 'waterways' and will be a good point to use. Other helpful tsubo include: SP 6 and 9, KID 1 and 3, LIV 3, 4 and 5, BL 22 and 31–4 (the four indentations in your sacrum), HT 8 and LI 6, which is helpful with eliminating upper-body oedema (*see* fig. 10.17).

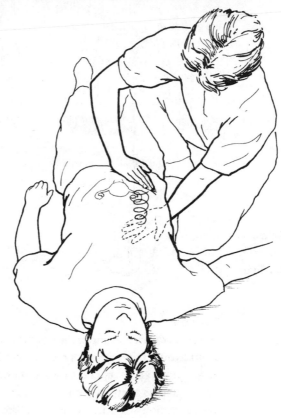

fig. 10.18 Ki projection into the ovaries

Ovarian Cysts

An ovarian cyst is a closed cavity or sac containing liquid or semi-solid material which develops in the ovary. Ovarian cysts may develop at any age and are rarely cancerous. As with fibroids, some ovarian cysts do not produce any symptoms at all, while others will show symptoms such as the swelling of the lower abdomen (without pain), difficulty in emptying your bladder, or a stinging, burning sensation when urinating. This is due to the cyst putting pressure upon the bladder itself. You might also have a brownish vaginal discharge, irregular periods or increased hairiness. The increased hairiness is due to the cyst producing a small amount of the male sex hormone, testosterone.

204

Treatment

We are once again looking at Ki stagnation. Follow the same recommenda-tion as under Fibroids on page 192. Treat your Spleen meridian in the leg; apply pressure to ST 17 and massage your nipples; apply pressure to GV 16 and the point between your eyebrows (GV 24.5); BL 20 tonifies Blood and Ki and 'softens hard masses'[5] (*see* fig. 10.17).

Get your partner to place their hand over the area of your ovary in your abdomen, with their other hand on the corresponding area of your back. 'Think' between the two hands, making a connection with the ovary in between and create warmth around it to help the Ki circulation (*see* fig. 10.18).

Premenstrual Tension (PMT)

This is the combination of various physical and emotional symptoms which occur in women one or two weeks before the onset of menstruation. It affects more than 90 per cent of fertile women at some time in their lives.

For a long time PMT was thought to be a psychological condition women used to gain sympathy. Today, however, it is recognized and defined as a 'dis-ease' and there are many theories about its cause. Hor-monal changes occurring throughout the menstrual cycle clearly influence PMT and progesterone therapy is very often the treatment of choice today, even if an imbalance between oestrogen and progesterone levels has not been consistently found.

Another possible cause for PMT is low blood sugar or hypoglycaemia, promoted by an unbalanced diet. Too much fat in your diet puts pressure on your liver and excess salt promotes fluid retention. If this is the case, you need to concentrate on establishing more regular eating habits. A good start would be to try to eat small meals throughout the day. Coffee and sugar deplete your body of the B vitamins, needed to keep your nervous system healthy and to stabilize your emotions. So exchange your cups of coffee for herbal teas and cut out the sugar. You can also take some vitamin B_6 supplements.

Yet another cause for PMT might be an imbalance in prostaglandins, causing the uterus to go into painful spasms. If there is an imbalance in the prostaglandins, your circulation will slow down and you will feel chilly and exhausted with pain and numbness in your hands and feet.

PMT is usually synonymous with mood swings and the most common emotional symptoms include irritability, tension, anger, depression and tiredness. It will often also affect a woman's self-esteem and you might feel

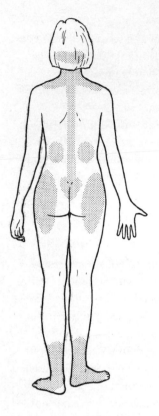

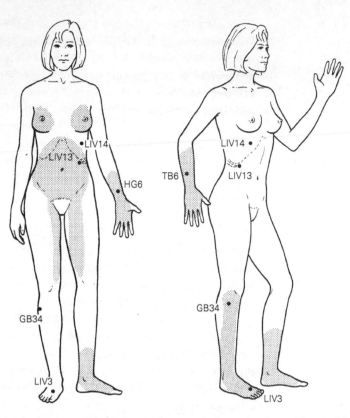

fig. 10.19
Premenstrual tension:
point location chart

'low', lacking concentration and control of your actions. Physical symptoms include headache, backache, lower abdominal pain and breast tenderness.

From an Oriental viewpoint, PMT symptoms are a sign of Blood and Ki stagnation. Ki is 'the commander' of Blood – when Ki stagnates, Blood coagulates. The build-up of tension within leads to all the different symptoms listed above.

The organ in charge of ensuring a smooth Ki flow throughout is the Liver. Its influence extends all over the body, to your intestines as well as your uterus. Moreover, it has a great influence on your emotional state: the smooth flow of Liver Ki ensures a 'smooth flow' of your emotional life. So when you are walking around feeling frustrated and angry, it is a sign that your Liver Ki is stagnated. If the Liver is functioning well and its Ki flowing smoothly, your emotional life will be happy and relaxed and you will find it easy to express your emotions and feelings.

How do you get to this state of being and how can you stimulate the Liver energy? Physical movement in any form is very beneficial, as the Ki gets stagnated in the joints and tendons very easily. You can choose to do some stretching to activate the Liver meridian (*see* the Liver stretch exercise on page 126–7) or dancing to music to release general stagnation. Kicking will help release tension in the hip area (one of the body areas which holds feelings like frustration and anger), as will hip rotations. Use your voice to express yourself vocally in combination with your physical movements; create sounds to release inner tension and free up your energy system.

Native Americans believed that women were most reflective and creative just prior to menstruation, so this is the time of the month to give the artistic part of yourself a chance to emerge and develop. Encourage this process by using visualization and/or affirmations (*see* Chapter 7).

Treatment
To disperse the Liver and regulate Ki, use the following tsubo: GB 34, LIV 3, 13 and 14, TB 6 and HG 6 – especially good for emotional imbalances (*see* fig. 10.19).

If you feel that your PMT symptoms are making you weak and over-emotional, you need to do something. Take a more responsible attitude and stop blaming yourself for not reaching a physical ideal. Learn to love yourself for the person you are and to not be so judgemental. If you become too hard on yourself, you will just make the situation worse and create more stress. Try to balance the amount of stress in your life and start a self-treatment programme using some of the suggestions above. Allow more time for yourself and your body and ask for help when you need it.

Prolapse
This is a condition where the uterus is displaced. Due to extreme stretching of the ligaments that hold the uterus in place, it descends from its normal position down into the vagina. Prolapse is most common among middle-aged women who have given birth, as childbirth can put lots of stress on these ligaments. A common symptom is the sensation of something pulling downwards in your pelvic region. If there is a severe prolapse, the uterus will be visible from the outside. Practising the pelvic floor exercises (*see* Chapter 8) is an excellent way of preventing a prolapse, especially after childbirth.

Treatment
Tsubo that 'raise the Ki' are: SP 6, GB 25 and 28, ST 29, 30 and 36 (*see* fig. 10.20). As Liver energy supports your muscular system, it will be helpful to stimulate the Liver meridian, paying special attention to LIV 3 and 8. Other beneficial tsubo include: KID 2, 5 and 6, and HT 8 (*see* fig. 10.20).

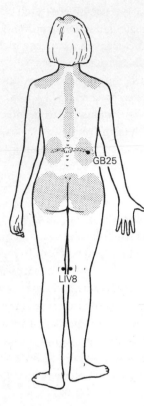
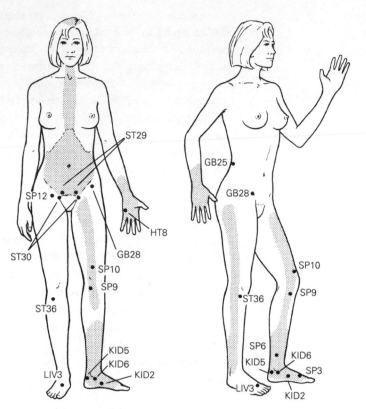

fig. 10.20
Prolapse/thrush: point
location chart

Thrush

This is an infection caused by the fungus *Candida albicans*. Usually you find this fungus in the vagina and mouth and its growth is kept in balance by natural bacteria in these organs. If for some reason your body's natural resistance to infections is decreased – through stress, exhaustion or antibiotic drugs, for example – the growth of the fungus is stimulated and you might get thrush. The most common symptoms are a thick, white vaginal discharge in combination with itching and irritation of the area. You might also have difficulty passing urine, but might on the other hand not have any of these symptoms at all. Thrush can also affect the mouth and produce creamy, yellowish patches inside your mouth, which can be very sore.

Treatment

This is a stagnant Blood condition with a lack of proper circulation of blood around the pelvis and genitals. As the Spleen assists the immune system and transportation of lymph, you need to tonify and treat your Spleen meridian in your legs. Focus on SP 3, 6, 9, 10 and 12 (*see* fig. 10.20).

Sea-salt baths are recommended, as is treating the area with natural yoghurt, both internally and externally. This will purify and cool down the hotness.

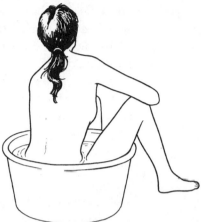

fig. 10.21 Hip bath

Alternatively, dry the leaves of daikon, radish or turnip until they are brown and brittle. Boil up a large pot of water (three to four litres/five to seven pints) and put the dry leaves in it. Let it simmer for 30–40 minutes until the water goes brownish. Add a handful of sea salt and prepare a hip bath for yourself. For this, preferably use a small tub, or pour the water (after filtering out all the leaves) into the bath tub. Add hot water so that the water reaches the level of your navel as you sit in it (*see* fig. 10.21). Keep the rest of your body covered up with towels. Take the bath as hot as possible and stay in it for 15 minutes, adding hot water if it cools down. If you should feel faint, get out of the bath immediately as it is too hot for you. Do this every day before going to bed for between seven and ten days. In Japan this is called a *Hiba Yu* bath and it is used extensively to maintain the reproductive organ health as it improves Blood movement.

Another remedy for improving the Blood movement in the genitals is to immerse a fresh tampon in a mixture of warm water and ginger juice – obtained from grating fresh ginger root in a ratio of 3:1 of water to juice. Insert the tampon as normal and change regularly. This may tingle for a few minutes to begin with but soon becomes comfortable.

Varicose Veins

To help blood return to the heart, the veins in your legs have a one-way valve system. If these valves collapse for some reason, it will increase the blood pressure in the veins and prevent proper drainage – this results in

Shiatsu for Women

enlarged or twisted superficial veins. They appear most often in the calves or on the inside of your legs. Standing for a long time or an excess of weight can be reasons for inadequate drainage (this is why pregnant women sometimes suffer from varicose veins). The hormonal changes during pregnancy also have a significant influence.

You should never apply pressure directly to varicose veins as it will be painful and there is some very slight risk of moving blood clots which may in turn reach the heart, causing a dangerous condition. Instead we advise you to use tsubo around the veins and other tsubo that will stimulate circulation. Regular exercise, such as walking or swimming, together with lying down with your feet up against the wall for 15 minutes daily, will also promote healthy circulation.

Treatment
Treat your Heart and Heart Governor meridians, paying special attention to the following tsubo: HT 1 (at the centre of your armpit), HT 7 and 9, HG 1, 6 and 9, and CV 17. Treating the Spleen meridian in your legs will also be beneficial as one of Spleen's function is to hold the Blood in place in the blood vessels: SP 6, 8, 9, 10 and 12 (*see* fig. 10.22).

fig. 10.22 Varicose veins: point location chart

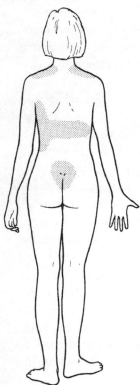

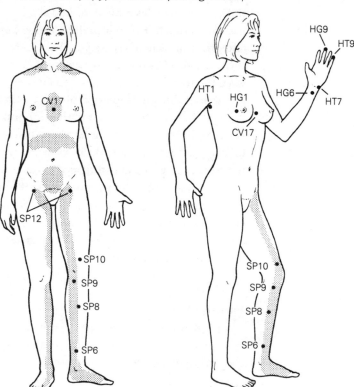

210

chapter 11

Self-Treatments for General Ailments

We are sure you will agree that, as a woman living in a busy world, it is not only your gynaecological health that is subjected to stress. Since you may suffer from other general ailments occasionally, here are some self-treatments to empower you.

Back, Neck and Shoulder Problems

Lower Back Pain

This is probably one of the most common complaints today. The human body is not built for the sedentary lifestyle we tend to live. To support a healthy spine you need to move and exercise your back. Sitting down at work, in your car or in buses, therefore, does not encourage a strong, healthy spine. Because we stand up and walk on two, rather than four limbs, we put a heavy load onto the lower back, so the vertebrae in the lumbar region are larger to be able to cope with this pressure. We also need to support the back with our muscles – well-toned back and abdominal muscles will give positive support to the skeletal structure. The only way to create strength in these muscles is to exercise them in different ways. Regular exercise and correct posture (*see* Chapter 3) will help prevent back pain.

It is very easy to get into the habit of adjusting your posture to release the pain you experience. However, this will only cause misalignments in your structure and can lead to referred pain in other body areas later on. In the case of severe pain, consult a qualified shiatsu practitioner and go for a course of treatments. Follow the suggestions below to ease mild back pain and practise the exercises between treatments for severe pain.

Treatment
Sea-salt baths (place a handful of sea salt in your bath water) will give some relief, as the hot water will help relax the muscles.

Use the tennis balls as described in Chapter 3 and work through the lower part of your spine, allowing the pressure to release the tension. Alternatively, get your partner to treat the whole Bladder meridian, as described in Chapter 4, focusing on the points in your sacrum: BL 31–4, 22, 23, 25, 27 and 28. Lie down on your front and support yourself with a cushion under your hip area, to bring your lower back more into flexion (rounded, not arched). The support from the cushion will open up the space between the different vertebrae in your lumbar area and allow for better circulation and energy flow (*see* fig. 11.1).

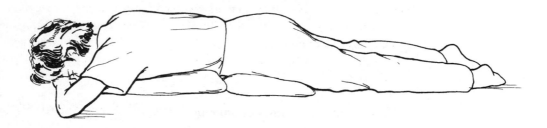

fig. 11.1 Flexed spine with the help of pillows

Other beneficial tsubo include: BL 50, 54 and 57, GV 4 and 1, GB 21 and 30 (*see* fig. 11.2). GB 30 can be treated by lying down on the floor and using the fist of your hand or a tennis ball into the point. Beneficial exercises include:

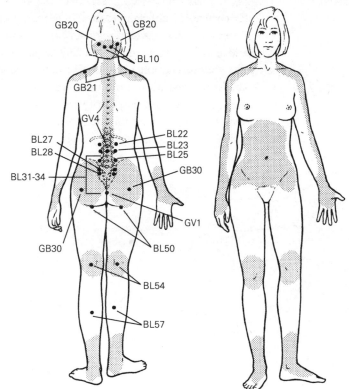

fig. 11.2 Lower back pain:
point location chart

Please note for reference to all illustrations:
All tsubo are bilaterally located on the body unless found on the midline.
Shaded areas indicate where to give general shiatsu treatment.

Relaxation Pose

- A good relaxation pose to help ease the pain in your lower back and also correct misalignments in your spine is to lie down on the floor with your lower legs resting on a chair (*see* fig. 11.3). This relaxes the lumbar area of your spine and straightens the whole spine. Gently push your lumbar region towards the floor to 'flatten' your spine.
- Close your eyes, allow your breathing to slow down, and visualize energy moving from the top of your spine down to the sacrum like a wave. Stay in this position for 10–15 minutes, two or three times a day.

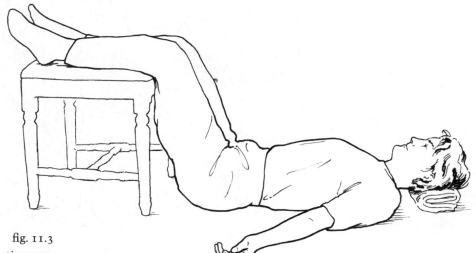

fig. 11.3
Relaxation pose

Sacral Massage and
Back Twist

- Follow up the above exercise with bringing the knees into your chest and gently pulling them towards your chest. Gently contracting your abdominal muscles, feel the sacrum against the floor and make circular movements with your knees. This will massage your sacrum and the sacroiliac joint and release tension in the area. Place your feet on the floor, keeping your knees bent. Take a deep breath in and relax your arms out to the sides.

- On the exhalation, allow both knees to drop over to the right side as you turn your head to the left, making sure your right shoulder stays on the floor. This will create a twist in your lower back and help to release any blockages in the area. Breathe in again and return to your starting position. Repeat to the other side and then another three times, going from one side to the other, coordinating your neck and leg movements (*see* fig. 11.4).

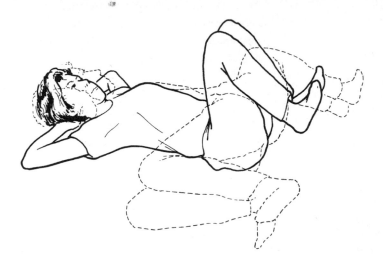

fig. 11.4 Back Twist

The Wave
- Stand with your feet shoulder-width apart, with bent knees. Place your hands just above the knees and straighten your back (*see* fig. 11.5). Sway back and look up to the ceiling.
- Bend your arms and slowly bring your upper body down towards the floor – making a deeper squat as you do so. Keep your eyes looking up to the ceiling until you can no longer see it. At this point, relax your head down and bring your back into flexion.
- Pull your abdominal muscles in and slowly roll up your spine from your sacrum, allowing the head to come up last. Lift the head up and straighten your spine. Move directly into the extension again and repeat the whole movement about ten times – imagine a wave rolling across your back, from the base of your spine to the top of your head.

This exercise will gently work through your whole spine, easing up blockages and improving energy movements throughout. While you are performing the exercise, you might find that some areas feel more in discomfort than others. If so, try to bring your attention to these areas and use your breathing to ease any pain.

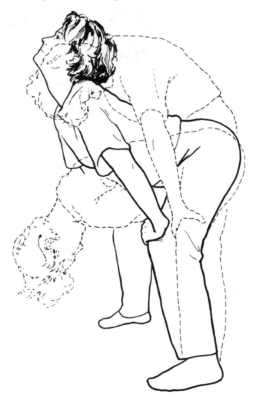

fig. 11.5 The Wave

Rotating
- Stay in the same position as above – feet shoulder-width apart, hands on your legs, just above the knees, and with a straight back. Breathe in and, on the exhalation, drop your left shoulder down between your legs (*see* fig. 11.6). Keep your elbows gently locked and look up to the ceiling over your right shoulder. Feel the twist in your spine.
- Take another deep breath in, return to starting position and drop your right shoulder down as you exhale. Repeat another three or four times on each side. Finish up by coming back to the starting position. Relax your upper body forwards. Walk your feet a bit closer together and slowly roll up your spine, until you come to a standing position.

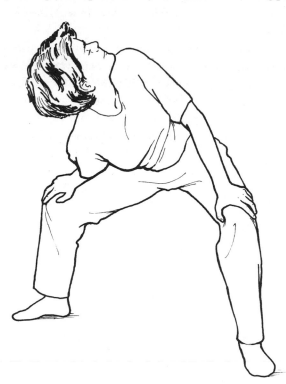

fig. 11.6 Rotating

After practising any exercises it is always good to finish by lying down in the Relaxation Pose again (*see* page 214). In combination with the above exercises, you also need to tune up your abdominal muscles. Refer to Chapter 9 under Strengthening Exercises.

Upper Back Pain

The upper part of the back often gets painful as a result of emotional stress. A slumped and collapsed posture often indicates sadness and depression – you feel unable to hold yourself upright and your shoulders fall forwards. The breathing becomes shallow and the energy level becomes low. Physical problems like colds, chest congestion, asthma or heart-related problems can also give rise to aches and pain in the upper back.

If the posture is slumped, you need to practise exercises that open up the chest area and create more space for you to breathe. The Wave, Sacral Massage and Back Twist and rotation exercises just described will all be very beneficial. Follow up with the exercises suggested below.

Opening Exercise for the Chest

- Stand with your feet slightly apart and lift your arms out to the sides to shoulder level. Bend your elbows and make lose fists with your hands. Inhale deeply and bring your arms back as much as possible, pushing your chest forwards. On the exhalation, bring your arms to a position in front of your chest.
- Cross your arms over and relax your head down, pressing the area between your shoulder blades backwards, so that you are rounding your upper back. Feel the muscles between your shoulder blades stretching. Empty your breath out completely, breathe in deeply again. Repeat the exercise four or five times (*see* fig. 11.7).

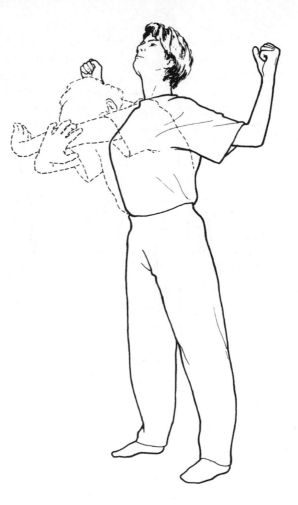

fig. 11.7 Opening
exercise for the chest

Treatment
Treat the Bladder meridian using the tennis balls (*see* Chapter 3) and get
your partner to apply pressure to the Bladder points situated between your
shoulder blades. Other beneficial tsubo are: GB 20 and 21 (*see* fig. 11.8
overleaf).

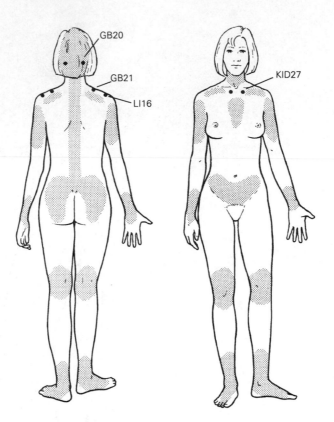

fig. 11.8 Upper back
pain: point location
chart

Neck and Shoulder Pain
Stiffness in the shoulders and neck is another common complaint arising
from stress. General worries, emotional problems and stress at home and
at work all add up and you feel the weight on your shoulders becoming
heavier and heavier, finally resulting in stiffness and aching. Of course
there could be an external force or injury causing the discomfort, or perhaps one of the External Pernicious Influences such as Wind prevalent.

Treatment
Gently tap your shoulder, using a loose fist, and get your partner to
squeeze and gently massage the top of your shoulders. Apply pressure to
the following tsubo to alleviate some of the pain: GB 20 and 21, BL 10 and
13, SI 4, 9, 10, 11, 12 and 15, TB 14 and 15, LI 15 and 16, GV 14, 15 and 16
(*see* fig. 11.9).

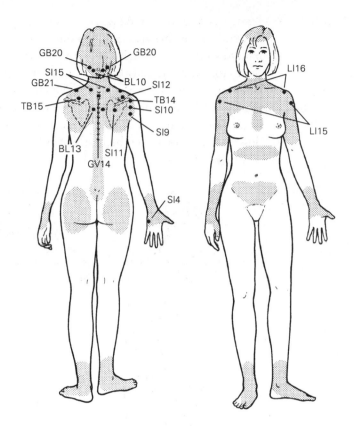

fig. 11.9 Neck and
shoulder: point location
chart

Do some general Do-In exercises for the upper body, chest and arms as described in Chapter 7, and treat the Small Intestine meridian using your thumbs. A good way of releasing tension in your neck and shoulders is to physically move them. Breathe in and lift your shoulders as high up towards your ears as you can. Hold your breath, keeping your shoulders on a level with your ears and feel the tension building up in the area. Breathe out, let go and allow your shoulders to just drop down. Feel the difference. Repeat a few times and then do circular movements with your shoulders. The opening exercises for the chest on pages 218–19 will also prove beneficial.

Because in shiatsu different body areas have energetic relationships, we can apply these relationships to help in the diagnosis and treatment of various conditions. The neck (cervical vertebrae) corresponds with the 'neck' of the thumbs and big toes – so to help your neck, massage your thumbs and big toes. It really works!

Neck Exercises • Straighten your back and lift your head up. Initiate the feeling of someone pulling you upwards from the top of your head. Slowly bring your
chin to your chest, stretching out the back of your neck. Clasp your
hands together and apply them to the back of your head. Drop your
elbows down and allow the weight of your arms to stretch out the
muscles in the back of your neck. Do not pull or force. Be very gentle
with yourself and gradually feel the area opening up. Relax your arms
down to the sides of your body and slowly bring your head back to the
centre (*see* fig. 10.10).

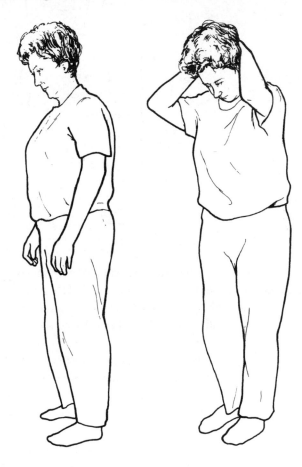

fig. 11.10 Stretching
exercise for the back of
the neck

- Looking forwards, bring your left ear towards your left shoulder. This will stretch out the right side of your neck. To improve on the stretch, bring your left hand to your right ear and allow the weight of your arm to further stretch the side of your neck. You can also press the palm of your right hand down towards the floor to increase the effect of the stretch. Once again, do not force these movements as you might easily pull a muscle, which will only cause more pain. Relax your arms and slowly bring your head back to the centre again. Repeat the stretch on the other side (*see* fig. 11.11).

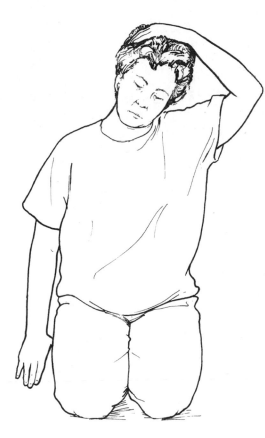

fig. 11.11 Side stretch for the neck

- Lift your chin up to the ceiling and drop your head back to stretch out the front of your neck. It is important to keep the rest of your back nice and erect. Bring your hands to your throat and gently stroke down the throat a few times to ease the tension in this area. Slowly bring your head back to the centre again (*see* fig. 11.12).

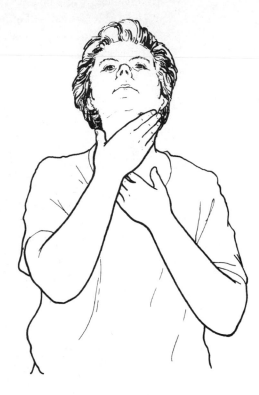

fig. 11.12 Stroking down
the throat

- Slowly turn your head to the right and then to the left. Repeat a few times and then drop your head to your right shoulder. From this position, make a half-circle with your head, bringing the chin to your chest and then slowly rolling the head over to the left side (ear to your shoulder) and back to the right side again. Repeat twice and then return to the centre with your head (*see* fig. 11.13).

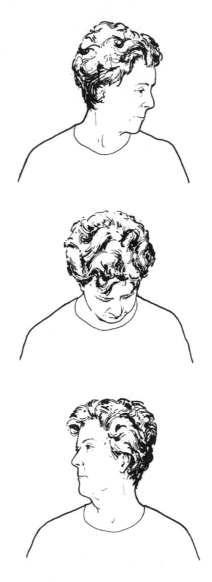

fig. 11.13 Head rolls from
side to side

- Finish by dropping your chin to your chest and slowly 'roll' down the spine. Relax your arms and gradually bring your upper body closer to the floor. Allow your knees to stay gently relaxed, then slowly 'roll' up again (*see* fig. 11.14).

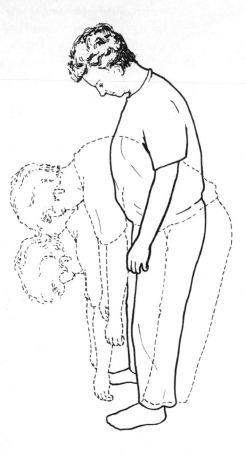

fig. 11.14 Rolling down
to the floor

Constipation

To prevent constipation, eat a well-balanced diet rich in fibres, grains and fresh vegetables. Chew your food well (50 times per mouthful) so that your food is in a liquid form before it reaches your stomach, and try to drink between meals rather than with your food. Make sure you get plenty of exercise and give yourself some Anpuku massage to stimulate the digestive process as follows:

Sitting down on the floor or in a chair, apply your fingers to the area just below your solar plexus. Spread your fingers out under the rib cage and take a deep breath in. Lean forwards from the waist and gently press your fingers up and under the ribs, as you breathe out (*see* fig. 11.15). At the end of the exhalation, relax completely and roll up again. Move your hands slightly to the left and repeat the same breathing, leaning forwards into the area underneath the left side of your rib cage. Exhale completely, relax and come up to sitting position again. Move your hands further down on the left-hand side of your abdomen, coming down to the area between your ribs and your hipbone. Repeat the same technique here, then move your hands down to the area inside your left hipbone and do the same thing. Continue to move your hands all the way around your abdomen in a clockwise direction, practising the same technique all the way around until you come back to your starting point. This exercise will gently massage your large intestine and give some support in the peristaltic movements of your bowels. (*See also* pages 62–3.)

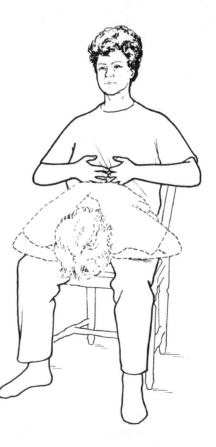

fig. 11.15 Anpuku

Treatment
Treat the Large Intestine meridian in your arms and apply pressure to the following tsubo: LI 4, 10 and 11, ST 25 and 36, SP 15, KID 3, LIV 1 and 3, and BL 25 (*see* fig. 11.16).

If you feel you need to induce a bowel movement, try the following home remedy: grate two tablespoons of radish pulp and mix with one tablespoon of soy sauce. Take two or three times a day, the first time on an empty stomach.

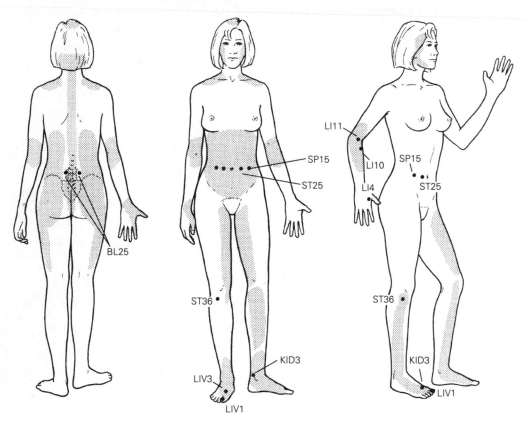

fig. 11.16 Constipation: point location chart

Diarrhoea

Three signs of good health are pleasant eating, pleasant sleep and pleasant bowel evacuation. Too many bowel movements per day or loose bowels indicate that something is not as it should be. Acute diarrhoea due to food poisoning, dysentery or overeating is usually of short-term duration and nothing to worry about. It can be considered as the body's reaction to clear out any toxins inside and, as such, very beneficial. But if the diarrhoea goes on for a long time or is very strong, there is a risk of dehydration, which can in turn cause chemical imbalances and lead to exhaustion. Long-term diarrhoea should therefore be checked by a doctor, shiatsu or other alternative health practitioner and given proper attention.

There are tsubo you can use to treat diarrhoea, but we strongly suggest some form of internal remedy in combination with your shiatsu (homoeopathy or herbal treatments, for example). If the diarrhoea is due to the intake of too much cold food – ice-cream, salads, raw fruit, fruit juices and generally too much liquid, for example – drink some ginger tea (boil three to five grams of ginger to make a tea).

Treatment
fig. 11.17 Diarrhoea: point location chart

Treat the Large Intestine meridian in your arms and apply pressure to the following tsubo: LI 1, 4, 10 and 11, ST 25, 34 and 36, CV 4, 5 and 12, BL 23 and 25, LIV 2, 6 and 13, SP 15, and GV 14 (*see* fig. 11.17).

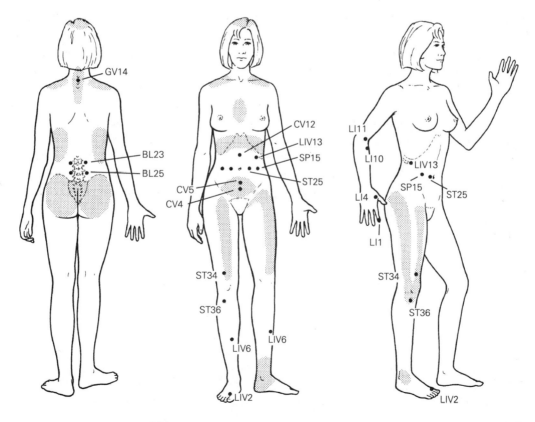

Headaches

Headaches can be due to many different causes and may be grouped into three basic categories according to K. Serizawa:[1]

- Irregularities in the blood vessels – pains such as migraine, throbbing pain and flashes in front of your eyes due to expansion of the blood vessels in your head.
- Muscular tension – due to work pressure, incorrect posture or external injury.
- Psychological matters and upsets.

In any of the above cases a full shiatsu treatment (as described in Chapter 4) will be the best start. It will relax you and improve the energy circulation throughout your body, so you will feel more balanced within. Headache is very often combined with neck and shoulder tension or even back pain. Refer to the treatments under these headings earlier in this chapter.

In addition to the full-body treatment, pay attention to the following tsubo: GV 16, 19, 20 and 24.5 (see fig. 11.18). You can gently massage these points yourself. With a light, finger pressure make small circular movements with your hand along the centre line of your head. After treating the GV channel, move your fingers to the outside (lateral) and treat the BL meridian on your head in the same way, focusing on BL 4, 7 and 10. Move towards your ears and bring your attention to the GB meridian. Use the same technique and pay special attention to GB 7, 12 and 20 (see fig. 11.18).

GB 21, on top of your shoulder, relieves whole body tension and will be helped by TB 5 and 17, and LI 4, 10 and 11. If you feel all your energy is in the upper part of your body and that you need to bring it down, apply pressure to ST 36, LIV 2 and 3 (see fig. 11.18).

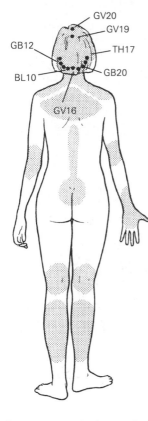
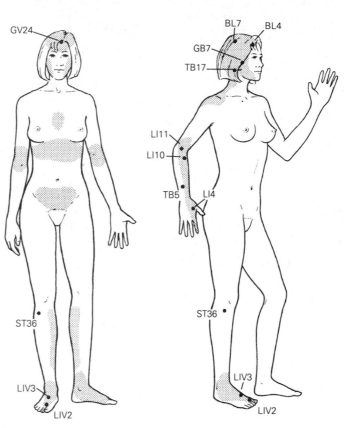

fig. 11.18 Headaches: point location chart

Indigestion

This refers to discomfort in the upper abdomen, brought on by stress or eating too much, too fast or food that is too fatty or spicy and therefore difficult to digest. All this brings on symptoms such as heartburn, abdominal pain, bloating or nausea (for treatment of these discomforts, see under each individual listed symptom). Although shiatsu treatment will help you in this case, adequate exercise as well as regular and wise eating habits are crucial for healing the problem.

Treatment

Eat smaller meals and avoid junk foods or 'heavy' foods full of spice or sauces. Treat the following tsubo: LI 4 and 10, ST 34 and 36, CV 1, 2 and 14 (*see* fig. 11.19, overleaf). Do the Anpuku abdominal massage described on pages 226–7.

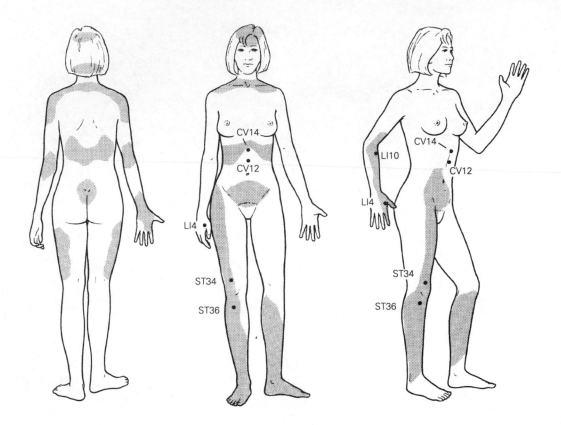

fig. 11.19 Indigestion: point location chart

Muscular Pain and Stiffness

This is a common condition which may arise from the usual lifestyle 'fatigue' syndromes including: poor diet not 'fuelling' your muscles (Spleen imbalance); lack of exercise not 'sparking' the fire of the muscles (Liver imbalance); excess thinking distracting attention away from your body (Spleen imbalance); overexercise stressing muscle fibres (Yang Excess); overworking causing Ki depletion and allowing Wind invasion.

Wind invades the Liver and creates muscular tension which is often active – that is, moves from one place to another. This is a more Yang disorder and will be relieved by Do-In exercises and self-massage. When the stiffness has become chronic, perhaps after an old injury, Blood stagnation and Ki Deficiency are leaving an area cold and stiff. This requires treating the whole system as well as the local area.

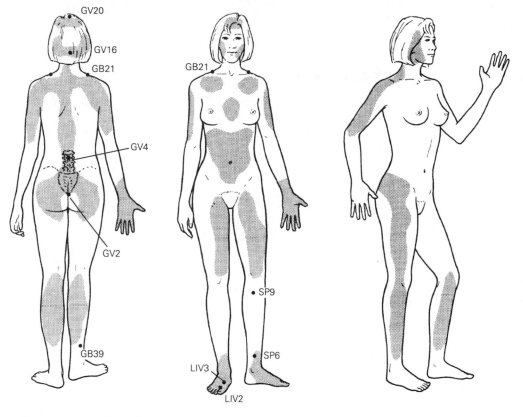

fig. 11.20 Muscular
pain and stiffness: point
location chart

Treatment

Treat the meridians of the Liver (for moving the Ki) and the Spleen (regulating the quality of the flesh). Give attention to the following tsubo: GV 20, 16, 4 and 2, LIV 2 and 3, SP 6 and 9, GB 21 and 39 (*see* fig. 11.20). Press tsubo in the local area to the pain – that is, any points which give relief. Attend to improving your diet and include leafy, green vegetables and reduce animal foods which can induce Liver Ki stagnation.

233

references

1. Introducing Shiatsu

1) Shunryu Suzuki, *Zen Mind, Beginner's Mind*, John Weatherhill Inc., New York and Tokyo, 1987.
2) *The Yellow Emperor's Classic of Internal Medicine – Simple Questions*, People's Health Publishing House, Beijing, 1979 (first published around 100 BC), pp. 4–6.

6. Assessing your Health with Shiatsu

1) Shaun de Warren, *The Health Handbook, Pearls to inspire healing*, Wellspring Publications, London, 1990.
2) Shaun de Warren, op. cit.
3) ibid.
4) As quoted in Susan Hayward, *You Have a Purpose, Begin It Now*, In-Tune Books, NSW Australia, 1990.
5) Susan Hayward, op. cit.
6) ibid.
7) Shaun de Warren, op. cit.
8) Shong Shu, *Practical Chinese Medicine*, Beijing Publishing House, Beijing (written between 659 and 627 BC).

References

9)   Dianne Connelly, *Traditional Acupuncture: The Law of the Five Elements*,
      The Centre for Traditional Acupuncture, Inc., Maryland USA, 1975, p. 11.

7. *Help Yourself to Health and Beauty*
1)   Ray Ridolfi, *The Shiatsu-Do Handbook*, 4th edition. British School of Shiatsu-
      Do Publications, London, 1995.
2)   Betty Edwards, *Drawing on the Right Side of the Brain*, J. P. Tarcher Inc., 1979.
3)   *What Doctors Don't Tell You*, The Wallace Press and Bryan Hubbard, vol. 6, no.
      5, August 1995.

10. *Self-Treatments for Common Gynaecological Problems*
1)   Bob Flaws, *Endometriosis and Infertility and Traditional Chinese Medicine*,
      A laywoman's guide, Blue Poppy Press, Boulder USA, 1989.
2)   The British Medical Association, *Complete Family Health Encyclopaedia*,
      Dorling Kindersley, London, 1990, p. 447.
3)   Bob Flaws, op. cit.
4)   *What Doctors Don't Tell You*, op. cit., vol. 4, no. 10.
5)   Arnie Lade, *Acupuncture Points, Images and Functions*, Eastland Press Inc.,
      Washington USA, 1989.

11. *Self-Treatments for General Ailments*
1)   Katsusuke Serizawa, *Tsubo, Vital Points for Oriental Therapy*, Japan
      Publications, New York and Tokyo, 1976.

glossary of some common shiatsu terms

Air Ki: a term used to describe the intake of oxygen.

Autonomic Nervous System: the involuntary nervous system, not under your conscious control.

Blood: a Fundamental Substance (*see* below) produced from the Ki of the Lungs, Spleen, Heart and Kidneys.

Deficiency: a term used to describe a condition of Ki depletion and may refer to a Deficiency of the body's normal Ki.

Essence: this is most commonly related to the Kidney Essence or the Spleen Essence, and indicates a purified or distilled fluid substance extracted from more dense materials.

Excess: a term used to describe a condition of Ki repletion. It may also be used to refer to an excess of a pathogenic influence such as Heat invasion.

Extraordinary Vessels: outside of the 12 traditional meridians, there are Extraordinary Vessels (energy channels) with a governing function for the 12 ordinary channels.

Fluids: these are the body fluids other than Blood and include sweat, saliva, gastric juices and urine.

Fundamental Substances: these are the primary foundations or building blocks for the production and storage of energy in all organic life. The Fundamental Substances are: Ki, Blood, Jing, Fluids and Shen.

Glossary of some Common Shiatsu Terms

Hara: the belly. Relates to the area between your ribs, hipbones and pubic bone. In Japan, the hara is traditionally thought of as your vital centre. It is the physical embodiment of the original Life centre.

Information: communication between the individual body systems to act as an integrated whole. 'Information potential' refers to our reserves which we can draw upon to fulfil our body's physical and spiritual needs. We often do not resource this potential efficiently and this becomes the basis for underachievement in our emotional, intellectual and spiritual bodies and may lead to physical illness. A catch phrase in our style of shiatsu is 'release your potential'.

Jing: this is the foundation substance necessary for all organic life forms to develop and mature. It is stored in the Kidneys. It is a combination of Pre- and Post-Heaven Essence.

Jitsu: a term used to describe observable energetic and physical manifestations of energy (Ki) movement. Jitsu means a fullness of energy or vitality (Excess).

Ki (Qi): this is the term used to describe your energy or Life Force. It is also the basis for the development of all phenomena from pre-molecular to physical and esoteric manifestations.

Kyo: a term used to describe observable energetic and physical manifestations of energy (Ki) movement. Kyo means an emptiness of energy or vitality (Deficiency).

Meridians (Channels): these are the energy channels or pathways along which Ki flows to all the body tissue.

Nutritive Ki (Gu Ki): this is the Ki derived from food and drink.

Pre-Heaven Essence: this is formed at the time of conception. This Essence, which nourishes the foetus during pregnancy, is what determines each individual's basic constitutional make-up, strength and vitality.

Post-Heaven Essence: the Essence which is refined and extracted from food and fluids after birth by the Stomach and Spleen.

Sedation: this involves movement and requires brushing, percussion, stimulating and strong stretching techniques to disperse the stagnant Ki and Blood, allowing these to move to areas of Deficiency.

Shen: a term used to describe the spirit or well-being of a person. The Shen is 'housed' in the heart.

Somatic Nervous System: the voluntary nervous system, the somatic nervous system produces conscious movement in the skeletal muscles.

Tonification: involves the attracting or gathering of energy back to an area deplete of Ki and Blood and requires holding techniques, waiting patiently for the Switch to occur. This may also be achieved with gentle stretches to relieve stiffness and improve mobility due to this form of 'emptiness' stagnation.

Tsubo: the pressure points found along the meridian pathways which are areas of concentrated electromagnetic charge.

237

Yang: a term used to describe energetic phenomena which may be used to describe a variety of manifestations of nature such as Fire, Sun, Sunlight, Masculine (*see* pages 7–8).

Yin: a term used to describe energetic phenomena which may be used to describe a variety of manifestations of nature such as Water, Moon, Shadow, Feminine (*see* pages 7–8).

Wei Ki: the defensive energy force of the body which is controlled by the Lung.

bibliography

Articles

Ray Ridolfi, 'Listening to the Moon, Reproductive Disorders and Shiatsu-Do' © 1994.
Ray Ridolfi, 'Shiatsu-Do, Pregnancy and Childbirth' © 1993.

Magazines

What Doctors Don't Tell You, The Wallace Press and Bryan Hubbard, various volumes.

Books

Cathryn Bauer, *Acupressure for Women*, The Crossing Press, California, 1987.

The British Medical Association, *Complete Family Health Encyclopaedia*, Dorling Kindersley, London, 1990.

Anne Charlish, *Your Natural Pregnancy, A Guide to Complementary Therapies*, Boxtree, London, 1995.

Dianne M. Connelly, *Traditional Acupuncture: The Law of the Five Elements*, The Centre for Traditional Acupuncture, Inc., Maryland USA, 1975.

Betty Edwards, *Drawing on the Right Side of the Brain*, J. P. Tarcher Inc., 1979.

Richard Feit and Paul Zmiewski, *Acumoxa Therapy Reference and Study Guide*, Paradigm Publications, Massachusetts USA, 1989.

Richard Feit and Paul Zmiewski, *Acumoxa Therapy Treatment of Disease*, Paradigm Publication, Massachusetts USA, 1990.

239

Bob Flaws, *Endometriosis and Infertility and Traditional Chinese Medicine, A laywoman's guide*, Blue Poppy Press, Boulder USA, 1989.

Bob Flaws, *The Path of Pregnancy*, Blue Poppy Press, Boulder USA, 1982.

Susan Hayward, *You Have a Purpose, Begin It Now*, In-Tune Books, NSW Australia, 1990.

Ted J. Kaptchuk, *Chinese Medicine, The Web that has no Weaver*, Rider & Company, London, 1983.

Michio Kushi, *Macrobiotic Home Remedies*, Japan Publications, Inc., New York and Tokyo, 1985.

Arnie Lade, *Acupuncture Points, Images and Functions*, Eastland Press, Seattle, Washington USA, 1989.

Giovanni Maciocia, *The Foundations of Chinese Medicine, A Comprehensive Text for Acupuncturists and Herbalists*, Churchill Livingstone, 1989.

Shizuto Masunaga, ZEN *Imagery Exercises, Meridian Exercises for Wholesome Living*, Japan Publications, Inc., New York and Tokyo, 1987.

Wataru Ohashi with Mary Hoover, *Natural Childbirth, The Eastern Way, A Healthy Pregnancy and Delivery Through Shiatsu*, Ballantine Books, New York, 1983.

Masahiro Oki, *Zen Yoga Therapy*, Japan Publications, Inc., Tokyo, 1979.

Paul Pitchford, *Healing with Whole Foods, Oriental Traditions and Modern Nutrition*, North Atlantic Books, California, 1993.

William Reed, *KI, A Practical Guide for Westerners*, Japan Publications, Inc., New York and Tokyo, 1986.

Ray Ridolfi, *Shiatsu-Do, The Handbook, Meridian personalities and tsubo location*, 3rd edition, British School of Shiatsu-Do, London, 1992.

Ray Ridolfi, *Alternative Health, Shiatsu*, Optima, London, 1990.

Swami Janakananda Saraswati, *Yoga, Tantra and Meditation*, Ballantine Books, New York, 1975.

Katsusuke Serizawa, *Tsubo, Vital Points for Oriental Therapy*, Japan Publications, New York and Tokyo, 1976.

Dr Miriam Stoppard, *Dr Miriam Stoppard's Pregnancy & Birth Book, the complete practical guide for all parents-to-be*, Dorling Kindersley, London, 1985.

Shunryu Suzuki, *Zen Mind, Beginner's Mind*, John Weatherhill Inc., New York and Tokyo, 1987.

William Tara, *Macrobiotic and Human Behaviour*, Japan Publication, Inc., New York and Tokyo, 1984.

Ilza Veith, *The Yellow Emperor's Classic of Internal Medicine*, new edition, University of California Press, 1972.

Shaun de Warren, *The Health Book, Pearls to inspire healing*, Wellspring Publications, London, 1990.

Dr H. Winter Griffith, *The Complete Guide to Symptoms, Illness & Surgery*, Equation, Wellingborough, 1987.

useful addresses

Finding a Practitioner
To locate a shiatsu practitioner in your local area contact:

The Shiatsu Society
31 Pulman Lane
Godalming
Surrey
GU7 1XY
Tel: 01483 860771

Studying Shiatsu
For enquiries about studying shiatsu in London and Branch Schools around the UK contact:

The British School of Shiatsu-Do (London)
6 Erskine Road
Primrose Hill, London
NW3 3AJ
Tel: 0171 483 3776
Fax: 0171 483 3804

Shiatsu for Women

Ray Ridolfi and Susanne Franzen give treatments at the British School of Shiatsu-Do (London) and in Bath at:

The Bath Natural Health Clinic
Alexander House
James Street West
Bath
BA1 2BP
Tel: 01225 313153

As a complementary learning tool to this book, you may be interested in purchasing the video, *Shiatsu-Do: The Way of Shiatsu*, from the British School of Shiatsu-Do (London). Tel: 0171 483 3776

index

(Figures in italics refer to illustrations.)

Index

245